BEAT PCOS

by Eating More COOKBOOK

A Food-First Approach to Reduce Cravings, Improve Insulin, and Lose Weight for those trying to conceive

GISELLE WRIGHT, BSN RN

Giselle Wright, BSN RN
Binnovate Publishers

Table of Contents

Introduction

Welcome to "Beat PCOS Weight By Eating More Cookbook"! This cookbook is designed to empower women navigating the challenges of Polycystic Ovary Syndrome (PCOS) through a food-first approach. Here, you will discover that nourishing your body with wholesome, delicious meals can help you manage your symptoms, reduce cravings, and improve your overall well-being. This is not just another diet; it's a lifestyle change that embraces the joy of eating while prioritizing your health.

Understanding PCOS

Polycystic Ovary Syndrome (PCOS) is a common hormonal disorder that affects approximately 1 in 10 women of reproductive age. It is characterized by a combination of symptoms that can vary widely among individuals. The condition is often associated with hormonal imbalances, insulin resistance, and inflammation, leading to a range of physical and emotional challenges.

Common Symptoms and Challenges Faced by Women with PCOS

Women with PCOS may experience a variety of symptoms, including:

- **Irregular Menstrual Cycles:** Many women with PCOS have infrequent or prolonged menstrual periods, which can complicate fertility.
- **Weight Gain:** Weight management can be particularly challenging due to insulin resistance, which can lead to increased fat storage.
- **Acne and Oily Skin:** Hormonal imbalances can cause skin issues, including acne and excessive oiliness.
- **Excess Hair Growth (Hirsutism)**: Many women experience unwanted hair growth on the face and body due to elevated androgen levels.
- **Thinning Hair**: Some women may notice hair thinning or male-pattern baldness.
- **Fertility Issues**: PCOS is one of the leading causes of infertility in women, making it a significant concern for those trying to conceive.

Understanding these symptoms is crucial for managing PCOS effectively. By recognizing the impact of PCOS on your body, you can take proactive steps toward improving your health and well-being.

The Importance of Nutrition

Nutrition plays a pivotal role in managing PCOS symptoms. Research has shown that dietary choices can significantly impact insulin levels, hormonal balance, and overall health. A well-balanced diet can help reduce inflammation, improve insulin sensitivity, and support weight management.

How Diet Impacts PCOS Symptoms, Cravings, and Insulin Levels

- **Insulin Resistance:** Many women with PCOS experience insulin resistance, which can lead to higher blood sugar levels and increased cravings for sugary and high-carbohydrate foods. A diet rich in whole foods, fiber, and healthy fats can help stabilize blood sugar levels and reduce cravings.
- **Hormonal Balance:** Certain foods can influence hormone levels. For example, incorporating foods rich in omega-3 fatty acids (like fatty fish and flaxseeds) can help reduce inflammation and improve hormonal balance.
- **Weight Management**: A nutritious diet can support weight loss or maintenance, which is crucial for managing PCOS symptoms. Studies have shown that even a modest weight loss of 5-10% can lead to significant improvements in symptoms and fertility.
- **Cravings**: Understanding the triggers behind cravings is essential for managing them. A diet that includes plenty of protein, fiber, and healthy fats can help keep you feeling full and satisfied, reducing the likelihood of unhealthy snacking.

Introduction to the "Eat to Beat" Philosophy

The ***"eat to beat"*** philosophy emphasizes the importance of nourishing your body with whole, nutrient-dense foods rather than restricting calories or following fad diets. This approach encourages you to focus on what you can eat rather than what you can't, promoting a positive relationship with food. By prioritizing foods that support hormonal balance and overall health, you can take control of your PCOS symptoms and enhance your fertility journey.

In this cookbook, you will find a variety of delicious recipes that align with the "eat to beat" philosophy, empowering you to make informed choices that support your health and well-being.

Chapter 1.

The Science Behind PCOS and Nutrition

Understanding Insulin Resistance

Insulin resistance is a condition where the body's cells become less responsive to the hormone insulin, which is responsible for regulating blood sugar levels. In women with Polycystic Ovary Syndrome (PCOS), insulin resistance is a common issue, affecting approximately 70% of those diagnosed with the condition.

Role of Insulin Resistance in PCOS

- **Hormonal Imbalance**: Insulin resistance leads to elevated insulin levels in the bloodstream (hyperinsulinemia). High insulin levels can stimulate the ovaries to produce more androgens (male hormones), such as testosterone. This hormonal imbalance can result in symptoms like irregular menstrual cycles, acne, and excessive hair growth.
- **Weight Gain:** Insulin resistance is closely linked to weight gain and obesity. When cells do not respond effectively to insulin, the body compensates by producing more insulin, which can promote fat storage, particularly in the abdominal area. This creates a cycle where weight gain exacerbates insulin resistance, making it even more challenging to manage PCOS.
- **Increased Risk of Metabolic Disorders**: Women with PCOS and insulin resistance are at a higher risk of developing metabolic disorders, including type 2 diabetes and cardiovascular disease. Managing insulin levels through diet and lifestyle changes is crucial for reducing these risks.

Managing Insulin Resistance

Dietary changes can significantly improve insulin sensitivity. A focus on whole foods, high-fiber carbohydrates, lean proteins, and healthy fats can help stabilize blood sugar levels and reduce insulin spikes. Regular physical activity is also essential, as exercise can enhance insulin sensitivity and support weight management.

The Connection Between Food and Hormones

The foods you consume can have a profound impact on your hormonal balance. Understanding how different foods affect your hormones is essential for managing PCOS effectively.

How Different Foods Affect Hormonal Balance

- **Carbohydrates**: Not all carbohydrates are created equal. Refined carbohydrates (like white bread and sugary snacks) can cause rapid spikes in blood sugar and insulin levels. In contrast, complex carbohydrates (such as whole grains, legumes, and vegetables) are digested more slowly, leading to more stable blood sugar levels.
- **Healthy Fats:** Incorporating healthy fats, such as those found in avocados, nuts, seeds, and olive oil, can help reduce inflammation and support hormonal balance. Omega-3 fatty acids, in particular, have been shown to improve insulin sensitivity and reduce androgen levels.
- **Protein**: Consuming adequate protein is crucial for managing cravings and maintaining muscle mass. Protein-rich foods can help stabilize blood sugar levels and keep you feeling full longer. Lean sources of protein, such as chicken, fish, legumes, and plant-based proteins, are excellent choices.
- **Fiber**: A high-fiber diet can help regulate blood sugar levels and improve insulin sensitivity. Foods rich in fiber, such as fruits, vegetables, whole grains, and legumes, can also promote gut health, which is increasingly recognized as important for hormonal balance.
- **Antioxidant-Rich Foods:** Foods high in antioxidants, such as berries, leafy greens, and nuts, can help reduce inflammation and oxidative stress, which are often elevated in women with PCOS.

The Role of Cravings

Cravings can be a significant challenge for women with PCOS, often leading to unhealthy eating patterns and weight gain. Understanding the underlying causes of cravings and how to manage them through diet is essential for effective PCOS management.

Understanding Cravings

- **Biological Factors**: Hormonal fluctuations, particularly in insulin and cortisol, can trigger cravings. For example, low blood sugar levels can lead to intense cravings for sugary or high-carbohydrate foods as the body seeks a quick energy source.
- **Emotional Factors**: Stress, anxiety, and emotional eating can also contribute to cravings. Women with PCOS may experience heightened stress due to their symptoms, leading to a cycle of emotional eating.
- **Nutritional Deficiencies**: Cravings can sometimes indicate nutritional deficiencies. For instance, a craving for chocolate may signal a need for magnesium, while a desire for salty snacks may indicate a need for sodium.

Managing Cravings Through Diet

- **Balanced Meals**: Eating balanced meals that include protein, healthy fats, and fiber can help keep you feeling full and satisfied, reducing the likelihood of cravings.
- **Mindful Eating**: Practicing mindful eating can help you become more aware of your hunger cues and emotional triggers. Take time to savor your food and listen to your body's signals.
- **Healthy Alternatives**: When cravings strike, opt for healthier alternatives. For example, if you crave something sweet, try fruit or a small piece of dark chocolate instead of sugary snacks.
- **Regular Meals**: Eating regular meals and snacks throughout the day can help stabilize blood sugar levels and prevent extreme hunger, which can lead to cravings.

Notes

Chapter 2.

Meal Planning for PCOS

Creating a Balanced Plate

Creating a balanced plate is essential for managing PCOS effectively. A well-balanced meal includes a variety of macronutrients—carbohydrates, proteins, and fats—along with plenty of vitamins and minerals. Here are some guidelines to help you build balanced meals that support your health.

Guidelines for Macronutrients and Portion Sizes

Carbohydrates

Aim for complex carbohydrates that are high in fiber, such as whole grains (quinoa, brown rice, oats), legumes (beans, lentils), and starchy vegetables (sweet potatoes, squash).
Portion size: Fill about ¼ of your plate with carbohydrates.

Proteins

Include lean protein sources to help stabilize blood sugar levels and keep you feeling full. Good options include chicken, turkey, fish, eggs, tofu, and legumes.
Portion size: Fill about ¼ of your plate with protein.

Healthy Fats

Incorporate healthy fats to support hormone production and reduce inflammation. Sources include avocados, nuts, seeds, olive oil, and fatty fish (salmon, mackerel).
Portion size: Fill about ¼ of your plate with healthy fats.

Vegetables

Fill the remaining half of your plate with non-starchy vegetables, such as leafy greens, broccoli, bell peppers, and zucchini. These are low in calories but high in nutrients and fiber.
Portion size: Aim for at least 2 cups of vegetables per meal.

Hydration

Don't forget to stay hydrated! Aim for at least 8 glasses of water per day, and consider herbal teas or infused water for variety.

Example of a Balanced Plate

Breakfast:
Scrambled eggs (protein) with spinach and tomatoes (vegetables) served with whole-grain toast (carbohydrates) and avocado (healthy fats).

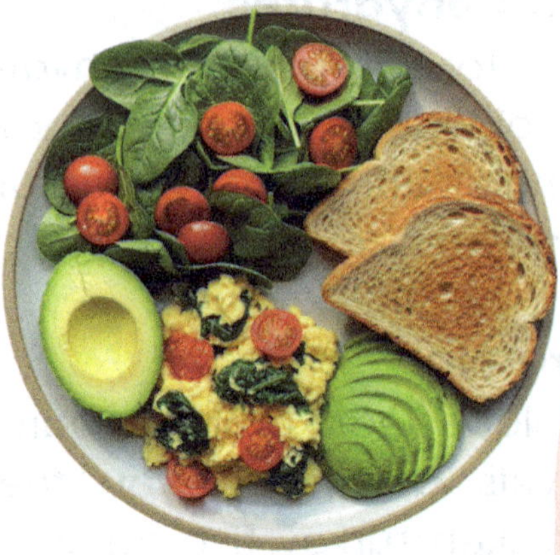

Lunch:
Quinoa salad (carbohydrates) with chickpeas (protein), mixed greens (vegetables), and olive oil dressing (healthy fats).

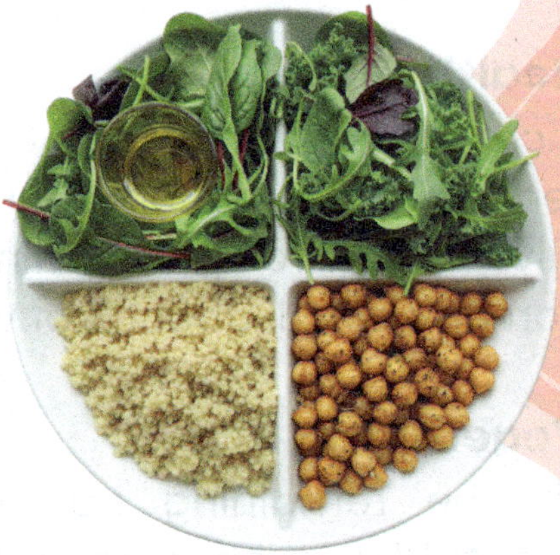

Dinner:
Grilled salmon (protein) with roasted sweet potatoes (carbohydrates) and steamed broccoli (vegetables) drizzled with olive oil (healthy fats).

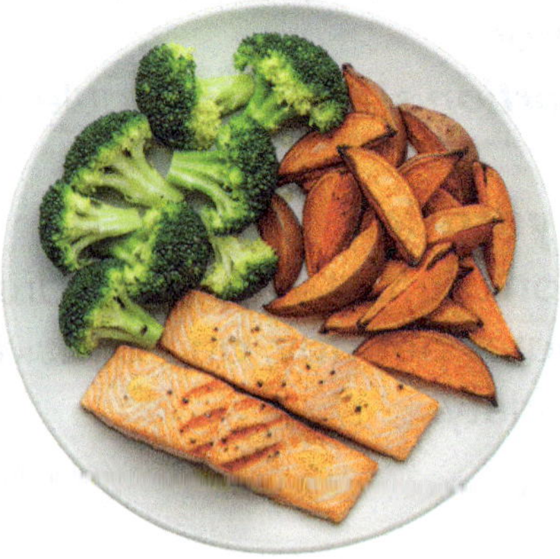

Meal Prep Strategies

Meal prepping can be a game-changer for managing PCOS. It helps you save time, reduce stress, and make healthier choices throughout the week. Here are some effective meal prep strategies:

- ***Plan Your Meals:***
  - Start by planning your meals for the week. Choose recipes that align with your dietary needs and preferences. Consider batch cooking staples like grains and proteins to use in various meals.
- ***Create a Shopping List:***
  - Based on your meal plan, create a shopping list to ensure you have all the ingredients you need. Stick to the perimeter of the grocery store where fresh produce, meats, and dairy are typically located.
- ***Batch Cooking:***
  - Dedicate a few hours each week to batch cook. Prepare large quantities of grains, proteins, and roasted vegetables that can be used in multiple meals. Store them in airtight containers in the fridge or freezer.
- ***Portion Control:***
  - Use portion control containers to divide meals into appropriate serving sizes. This can help you avoid overeating and make it easier to grab a healthy meal on the go.
- ***Snack Prep:***
  - Prepare healthy snacks in advance, such as cut-up vegetables, hummus, or energy balls. Having healthy options readily available can help curb cravings and prevent unhealthy snacking.
- ***Stay Flexible:***
  - While meal prepping is helpful, it's essential to stay flexible. Life can be unpredictable, so be open to adjusting your meals as needed.

Notes

Chapter 3.

PCOS - Friendly

Breakfast Recipes

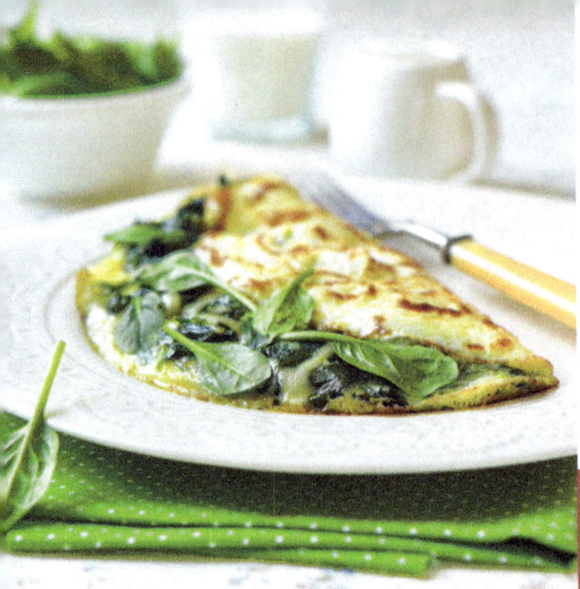

Spinach and Feta Omelette

SERVING SIZE
Serves 1

INGREDIENTS

- 2 large eggs
- 1 cup fresh spinach, chopped
- 1/4 cup feta cheese, crumbled (dairy-free if needed)
- 1 tablespoon olive oil
- Salt and pepper to taste
- *Optional*
  Fresh herbs (like parsley or dill) for garnish

DIRECTIONS

1. **Prepare Ingredients:** In a bowl, whisk the eggs with salt and pepper until weii combined.
2. **Sauté Spinach:** In a non-stick skillet, heat olive oil over medium heat. Add the chopped spinach and sauté for about 1-2 minutes until wilted.
3. **Add Eggs:** Pour the whisked eggs over the sautéed spinach, tilting the pan to ensure even coverage. Cook for about 2-3 minutes, or until the edges start to set.
4. **Add Feta:** Sprinkle the crumbled feta cheese over one half of the omelette.
5. **Fold Omelette:** Once the eggs are mostly set, carefully fold the omelette in half over the feta. Cook for an additional 1-2 minutes until the cheese is slightly melted and the eggs are fully cooked.
6. **Serve:** Slide the omelette onto a plate and garnish with fresh herbs if desired. Serve warm.

Nutrition Information (Per Serving)

Calories	250
Protein	18g
Carbohydrates	2g
Dietary Fiber	1g
Sugars	1g
Fat	20g
Saturated Fat	5g

"You are not alone."

QUICK NOTES

TIPS FOR CUSTOMIZATION

- **Add Veggies:** Include other vegetables like bell peppers, onions, or mushrooms for added nutrition.
- **Spice it Up:** Add a pinch of red pepper flakes or hot sauce for extra heat.
- **Cheese Variations:** Substitute feta with goat cheese or nutritional yeast for a dairy-free option.

Why is this recipe good for PCOS?

This spinach and feta omelette is high in protein and healthy fats, which help regulate blood sugar levels and promote satiety. The spinach provides essential vitamins and minerals, while the feta adds flavor and calcium. This dish is low in carbohydrates and nutrient-dense, making it a great option for women managing PCOS.

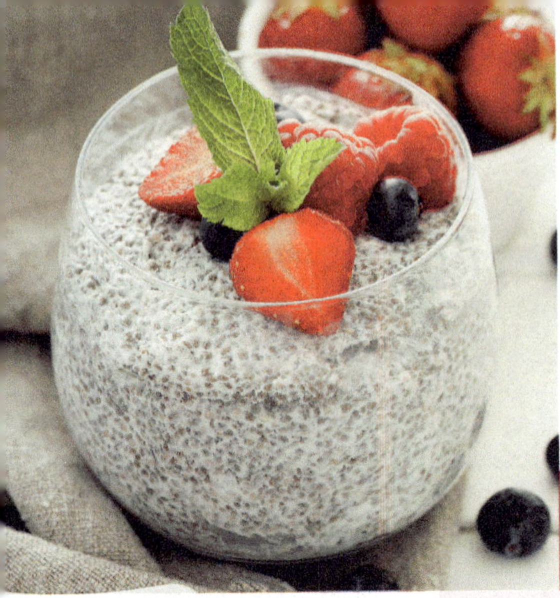

Chia Seed Pudding with Almond Milk and Berries

SERVING SIZE
Serves 1

INGREDIENTS

- 1/4 cup chia seeds
- 1 cup unsweetened almond milk (or any dairy-free milk)
- 1 tablespoon maple syrup or a low-carb sweetener (like stevia or erythritol) to taste
- 1/2 teaspoon vanilla extract (optional)
- 1/2 cup mixed berries (fresh or frozen, such as strawberries, blueberries, or raspberries)
- *Optional* Nuts or seeds for topping

DIRECTIONS

1. **Mix Ingredients:** In a bowl or jar, combine chia seeds, almond milk, maple syrup (or sweetener), and vanilla extract (if using). Stir well to ensure the chia seeds are evenly distributed.
2. **Refrigerate:** Cover the bowl or jar and refrigerate for at least 4 hours or overnight. The chia seeds will absorb the liquid and thicken to a pudding-like consistency.
3. **Stir and Serve:** After chilling, stir the pudding to break up any clumps. Top with mixed berries and nuts or seeds if desired before serving.

Nutrition Information (Per Serving)

Calories	250
Protein	6g
Carbohydrates	20g
Dietary Fiber	15g
Sugars	5g
Fat	16g
Saturated Fat	1g

"Your journey is unique."

QUICK NOTES

TIPS FOR CUSTOMIZATION

- **Add Flavor:** Mix in a pinch of cinnamon or cocoa powder for different flavor profiles.
- **Fruit Options:** Use any seasonal fruits or your favorite berries for topping.
- **Nut Milk Alternatives:** Substitute almond milk with coconut milk or any other dairy-free milk of your choice.

Why is this recipe good for PCOS?

Chia seeds are an excellent source of omega-3 fatty acids, fiber, and protein, which help regulate blood sugar levels and promote satiety. The high fiber content aids in digestion and can help manage weight, which is beneficial for women with PCOS. This pudding is low in refined sugars and high in nutrients, making it a delicious and healthy breakfast or snack option.

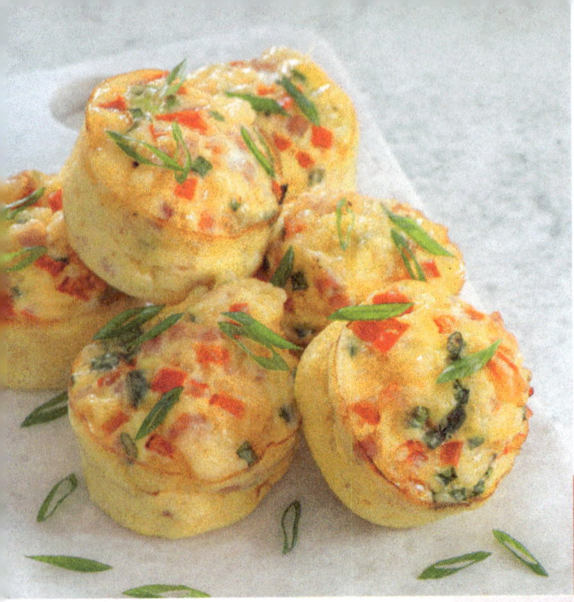

Egg Muffins with Bell Peppers and Turkey Bacon

SERVING SIZE
Serves 3 (2 muffins per serving)

INGREDIENTS

- 6 large eggs
- 1/2 cup bell peppers, diced (any color)
- 1/2 cup cooked turkey bacon, chopped
- 1/4 cup onion, finely diced
- 1/2 teaspoon garlic powder
  Salt and pepper to taste
- *Optional*
  1/4 cup shredded cheese (dairy-free if needed) for topping
- *Optional*
  Fresh herbs (like parsley or chives) for garnish

DIRECTIONS

1. **Preheat Oven:** Preheat your oven to 350ºF (175ºC). Grease a muffin tin with cooking spray or line with silicone muffin cups.
2. **Prepare Egg Mixture:** In a large bowl, whisk together the eggs, garlic powder, salt, and pepper until well combined.
3. **Add Fillings:** Stir in the diced bell peppers, chopped turkey bacon, and diced onion until evenly distributed.
4. **Fill Muffin Tin:** Pour the egg mixture evenly into the prepared muffin tin, filling each cup about 3/4 full. If using, sprinkle shredded cheese on top of each muffin.
5. **Bake:** Bake in the preheated oven for 18-20 minutes, or until the egg muffins are set and lightly golden on top.
6. **Cool and Serve:** Allow the muffins to cool for a few minutes before removing them from the tin. Serve warm or store in the refrigerator for later.

Nutrition Information (Per Serving)

Calories	200
Protein	18g
Carbohydrates	4g
Dietary Fiber	1g
Sugars	1g
Fat	12g
Saturated Fat	3g

"Embrace your strength."

QUICK NOTES

TIPS FOR CUSTOMIZATION

- **Add Veggies:** Include additional vegetables like spinach, zucchini, or mushrooms for added nutrition.
- **Spice it Up:** Add red pepper flakes or hot sauce for a spicy kick.
- **Herb Variations:** Experiment with fresh herbs like basil or cilantro for added flavor.

Why is this recipe good for PCOS?

These egg muffins are high in protein and healthy fats, which help regulate blood sugar levels and promote satiety. The combination of vegetables provides essential vitamins and minerals, while turkey bacon adds lean protein without excess fat. This recipe is low in carbohydrates and can be made in advance, making it a convenient and nutritious option for women managing PCOS.

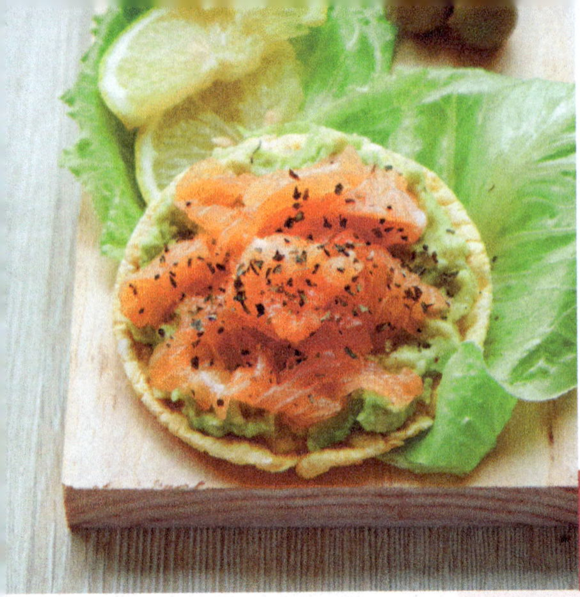

Avocado and Smoked Salmon on Rice Cakes

SERVING SIZE
Serves 1

INGREDIENTS

- 2 plain rice cakes (gluten-free if needed)
- 1 ripe avocado
- 4 ounces smoked salmon
- Juice of 1/2 lemon
- Salt and pepper to taste
- *Optional* Capers for garnish
- *Optional* Fresh dill or chives for garnish

DIRECTIONS

1. **Prepare Avocado:** In a bowl, mash the avocado with a fork. Add lemon juice, salt, and pepper to taste, mixing until well combined.
2. **Assemble Rice Cakes:** Spread a generous layer of the mashed avocado on each rice cake.
3. **Top with Salmon:** Place slices of smoked salmon on top of the avocado spread.
4. **Garnish:** If desired, garnish with capers and fresh dill or chives for added flavor.
5. **Serve:** Enjoy immediately as a healthy snack or light meal.

Nutrition Information (Per Serving)

Calories	350
Protein	20g
Carbohydrates	30g
Dietary Fiber	8g
Sugars	1g
Fat	20g
Saturated Fat	3g

"You are enough."

QUICK NOTES

TIPS FOR CUSTOMIZATION

- **Add Flavor:** Mix in a dash of garlic powder or red pepper flakes to the avocado for extra flavor.
- **Vegetable Variations:** Include sliced cucumbers or radishes for added crunch and nutrition.
- **Nut Variations:** Top with chopped nuts or seeds for added texture.

Why is this recipe good for PCOS?

This dish is rich in healthy fats from avocado and protein from smoked salmon, which help regulate blood sugar levels and promote satiety. The fiber from rice cakes and vegetables aids in digestion and can help manage weight, which is beneficial for women with PCOS. This recipe is quick to prepare, nutritious, and perfect for a satisfying snack or light meal.

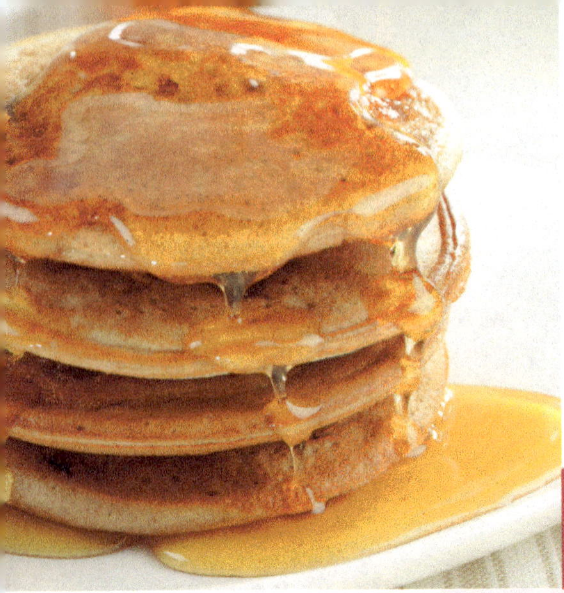

Coconut Flour Pancakes with Sugar-Free Maple Syrup

SERVING SIZE
Serves 1 (makes about 2-3 pancakes)

INGREDIENTS

- 1/4 cup coconut flour
- 1/4 teaspoon baking powder
- 1/4 teaspoon salt
- 3 large eggs
- 1/4 cup unsweetened almond milk (or any dairy-free milk)
- 1 tablespoon coconut oil, melted (plus extra for cooking)
- 1 teaspoon vanilla extract
- *Optional* Sugar-free maple syrup for serving

DIRECTIONS

1. **Mix Dry Ingredients:** In a bowl, combine coconut flour, baking powder, and salt. Mix well to ensure there are no lumps.
2. **Combine Wet Ingredients:** In a separate bowl, whisk together the eggs, almond milk, melted coconut oil, and vanilla extract until smooth.
3. **Combine Mixtures:** Gradually add the wet ingredients to the dry ingredients, stirring until well combined. Let the batter sit for about 5 minutes to thicken.
4. **Cook Pancakes:** Heat a non-stick skillet over medium heat and add a small amount of coconut oil. Pour about 1/4 cup of batter onto the skillet for each pancake. Cook for 2-3 minutes, or until bubbles form on the surface, then flip and cook for an additional 1-2 minutes until golden brown.
5. **Serve:** Stack the pancakes on a plate and serve warm with sugar-free maple syrup, if desired.

Nutrition Information (Per Serving)

Calories	300
Protein	12g
Carbohydrates	20g
Dietary Fiber	10g
Sugars	2g
Fat	20g
Saturated Fat	10g

"Every day is a new beginning."

QUICK NOTES

TIPS FOR CUSTOMIZATION

- **Add Flavor:** Mix in cinnamon or nutmeg for added flavor.
- **Fruit Toppings:** Top with fresh berries or sliced bananas for natural sweetness.
- **Nut Variations:** Add chopped nuts or seeds to the batter for extra crunch.

Why is this recipe good for PCOS?

Coconut flour is high in fiber and low in carbohydrates, making it a great option for managing blood sugar levels. The healthy fats from coconut oil and the protein from eggs help promote satiety and hormone balance. This pancake recipe is a delicious, low-carb alternative to traditional pancakes, allowing women with PCOS to enjoy a satisfying breakfast without the guilt.

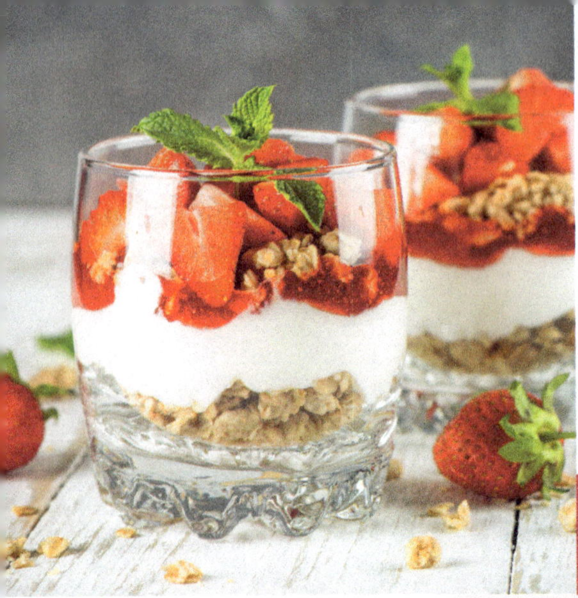

Greek Yogurt Parfait with Nuts and Seeds

SERVING SIZE
Serves 1

INGREDIENTS

- 1 cup plain Greek yogurt (dairy-free if needed)
- 1/4 cup mixed nuts (such as almonds, walnuts, and pecans), chopped
- 2 tablespoons seeds (such as chia seeds, flaxseeds, or pumpkin seeds)
- 1/2 cup mixed berries (fresh or frozen, such as strawberries, blueberries, or raspberries)
- 1 tablespoon honey or a low-carb sweetener (like stevia or erythritol) to taste
- *Optional*
  1/2 teaspoon vanilla extract for added flavor

DIRECTIONS

1. **Prepare Yogurt Base:** In a bowl, mix the Greek yogurt with honey (or sweetener) and vanilla extract (if using) until well combined.
2. **Layer Ingredients:** In a serving glass or bowl, layer half of the yogurt mixture at the bottom. Add half of the mixed berries, followed by half of the chopped nuts and seeds.
3. **Repeat Layers:** Add another layer of the remaining yogurt mixture, followed by the rest of the berries, nuts, and seeds.
4. **Serve:** Enjoy immediately as a nutritious breakfast or snack.

Nutrition Information (Per Serving)

Calories	350
Protein	25g
Carbohydrates	30g
Dietary Fiber	8g
Sugars	10g
Fat	18g
Saturated Fat	3g

"Believe in your power."

QUICK NOTES

TIPS FOR CUSTOMIZATION

- **Add Flavor:** Mix in a pinch of cinnamon or nutmeg for extra flavor.
- **Fruit Options:** Use any seasonal fruits or your favorite berries for topping.
- **Nut Variations:** Substitute nuts with seeds or granola for different textures.

Why is this recipe good for PCOS?

This Greek yogurt parfait is high in protein, which helps regulate blood sugar levels and promotes satiety. The combination of nuts and seeds provides healthy fats and fiber, which are beneficial for hormone balance. The berries add antioxidants and vitamins, making this a nutritious and satisfying option for women managing PCOS.

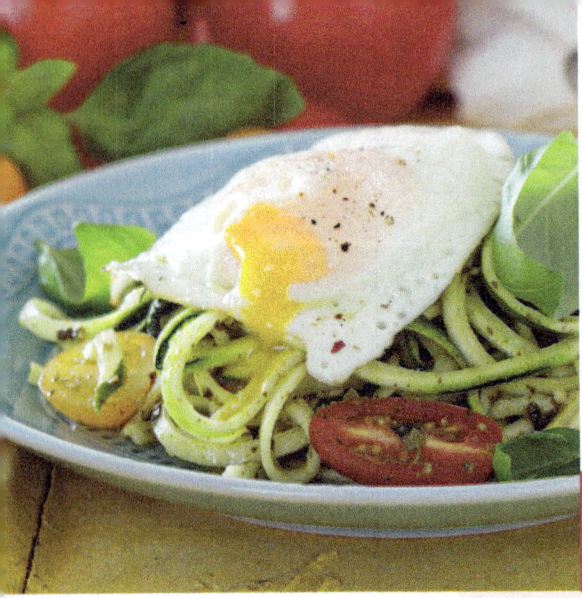

Zucchini Noodles with Scrambled Eggs and Cherry Tomatoes

SERVING SIZE
Serves 1

INGREDIENTS

- 2 medium zucchinis, spiralized into noodles
- 2 large eggs
- 1 cup cherry tomatoes, halved
- 1 tablespoon olive oil
- 1 clove garlic, minced
- Salt and pepper to taste
- *Optional*
  Fresh basil or parsley for garnish
- *Optional*
  Nutritional yeast for a cheesy flavor

DIRECTIONS

1. **Prepare Zucchini Noodles:** Spiralize the zucchinis into noodles and set aside.
2. **Sauté Garlic and Tomatoes:** In a large skillet, heat olive oil over medium heat. Add minced garlic and sauté for about 30 seconds until fragrant. Add the halved cherry tomatoes and cook for about 3-4 minutes, until they start to soften.
3. **Add Zucchini Noodles:** Add the spiralized zucchini noodles to the skillet and cook for an additional 2-3 minutes, stirring gently until the noodles are tender but still slightly crisp.
4. **Scramble the Eggs:** In a bowl, whisk the eggs with salt and pepper. Push the zucchini noodles and tomatoes to one side of the skillet and pour the eggs into the other side. Scramble the eggs until fully cooked, then mix them with the zucchini noodles and tomatoes.
5. **Serve:** Remove from heat and garnish with fresh herbs and nutritional yeast if desired. Serve immediately.

Nutrition Information (Per Serving)

Calories	250
Protein	12g
Carbohydrates	10g
Dietary Fiber	4g
Sugars	4g
Fat	20g
Saturated Fat	3g

"You are resilient."

QUICK NOTES

TIPS FOR CUSTOMIZATION

- **Add Protein:** Include cooked chicken, turkey, or tofu for extra protein.
- **Spice it Up:** Add red pepper flakes or hot sauce for a spicy kick.
- **Vegetable Variations:** Incorporate other vegetables like bell peppers, spinach, or onions for added nutrition.

Why is this recipe good for PCOS?

Zucchini noodles are low in carbohydrates and high in fiber, making them an excellent choice for managing blood sugar levels. The combination of eggs provides high-quality protein and healthy fats, which are essential for hormone balance. This dish is nutrient-dense and satisfying, making it a great option for women with PCOS looking for a healthy and delicious meal.

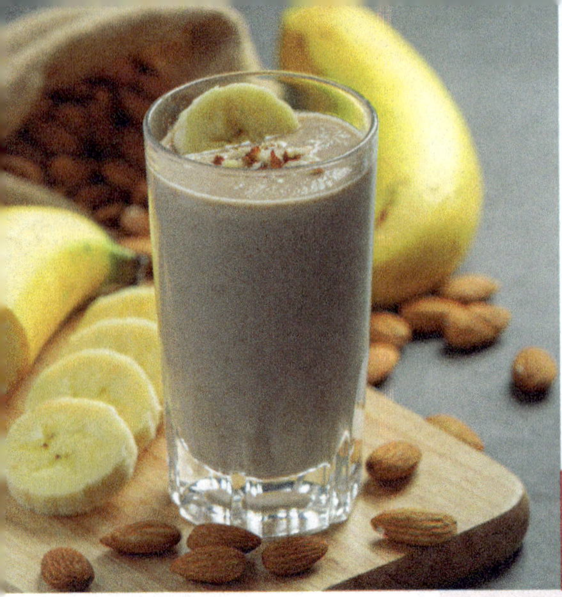

Almond Butter and Banana Smoothie

SERVING SIZE
Serves 1

INGREDIENTS

- 1 medium ripe banana
- 2 tablespoons almond butter
- 1 cup unsweetened almond milk
- 1 tablespoon chia seeds (optional)
- 1/2 teaspoon cinnamon (optional)
- Ice cubes (optional, for a chilled smoothie)

DIRECTIONS

1. **Combine Ingredients:** In a blender, add the banana, almond butter, unsweetened almond milk, chia seeds (if using), and cinnamon (if using).
2. **Blend:** Blend on high speed until smooth and creamy. If you prefer a thicker smoothie, add a few ice cubes and blend again until desired consistency is reached.
3. **Serve:** Pour the smoothie into a glass and enjoy immediately.

Nutrition Information (Per Serving)

Calories	350
Protein	10g
Carbohydrates	30g
Dietary Fiber	8g
Sugars	12g
Fat	22g
Saturated Fat	2g

"Your health matters."

QUICK NOTES

TIPS FOR CUSTOMIZATION

- **Add Greens:** Toss in a handful of spinach or kale for added nutrients without altering the flavor significantly.
- **Protein Boost:** Add a scoop of protein powder for an extra protein boost.
- **Flavor Variations:** Experiment with different nut butters, such as cashew or peanut butter, for variety.

Why is this recipe good for PCOS?

This smoothie is rich in healthy fats from almond butter, which helps regulate blood sugar levels and promotes satiety. The banana provides natural sweetness and potassium, while chia seeds add fiber and omega-3 fatty acids, which are beneficial for hormone balance. This nutrient-dense smoothie is a quick and easy breakfast option for women managing PCOS, providing sustained energy throughout the morning.

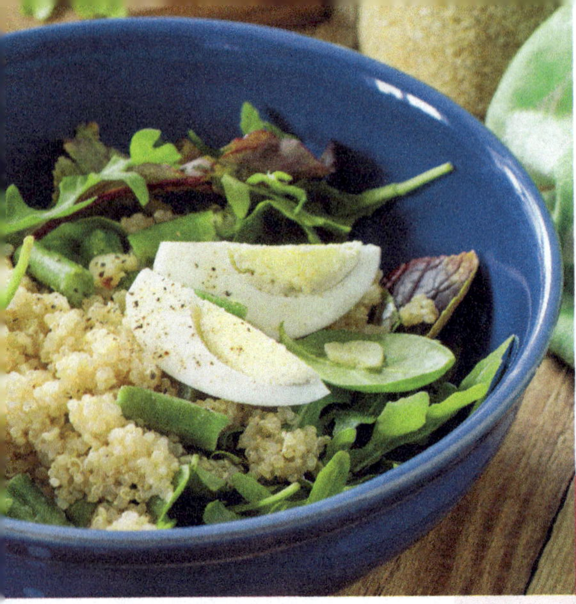

Savory Quinoa Breakfast Bowl with Spinach and Eggs

SERVING SIZE
Serves 1

INGREDIENTS

- 1/2 cup cooked quinoa
- 2 large eggs
- 1 cup fresh spinach, chopped
- 1 tablespoon olive oil
- 1/4 teaspoon garlic powder
  Salt and pepper to taste
- *Optional*
  1/4 avocado, sliced, for topping
- *Optional*
  Hot sauce for serving

DIRECTIONS

1. **Prepare Quinoa:** If you haven't already, cook quinoa according to package instructions. Allow it to cool or use chilled quinoa for a refreshing breakfast bowl.
2. **Sauté Spinach:** In a skillet, heat olive oil over medium heat. Add the chopped spinach and garlic powder, and sauté for about 2-3 minutes until the spinach is wilted. Season with salt and pepper to taste.
3. **Cook Eggs:** In a separate pan, cook the eggs to your liking (scrambled, fried, or poached).
   Assemble Bowl: In a serving bowl, layer the cooked quinoa, sautéed spinach, and cooked eggs.
4. **Serve:** Top with sliced avocado if desired and drizzle with hot sauce for extra flavor. Enjoy warm.

Nutrition Information (Per Serving)

Calories	350
Protein	20g
Carbohydrates	30g
Dietary Fiber	8g
Sugars	2g
Fat	18g
Saturated Fat	3g

"Take it one step at a time."

QUICK NOTES

TIPS FOR CUSTOMIZATION

- **Add Veggies:** Include other vegetables like bell peppers, tomatoes, or mushrooms for added nutrition.
- **Spice it Up:** Add red pepper flakes or your favorite seasoning blend for extra flavor.
- **Herb Variations:** Experiment with fresh herbs like basil or cilantro for added freshness.

Why is this recipe good for PCOS?

This savory quinoa breakfast bowl is high in protein and fiber, which help regulate blood sugar levels and promote satiety. The combination of quinoa and eggs provides essential nutrients, while the healthy fats from olive oil and avocado support hormone balance. This dish is nutrient-dense and satisfying, making it a great option for women managing PCOS.

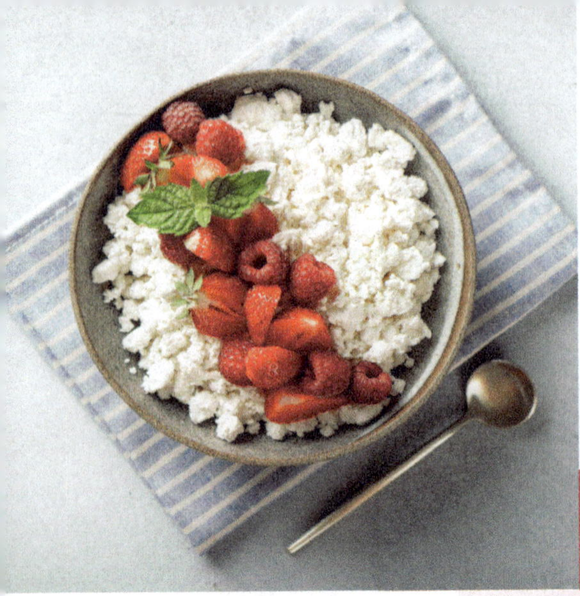

Cottage Cheese Bowl with Berries and Flaxseeds

SERVING SIZE
Serves 1

INGREDIENTS

- 1 cup cottage cheese (dairy-free if needed)
- 1/2 cup mixed berries (fresh or frozen, such as strawberries, blueberries, or raspberries)
- 2 tablespoons ground flaxseeds
- 1 tablespoon honey or a low-carb sweetener (like stevia or erythritol) to taste
- *Optional* 1/4 teaspoon cinnamon for added flavor
- *Optional* Chopped nuts or seeds for topping

DIRECTIONS

1. **Prepare Cottage Cheese:** In a bowl, add the cottage cheese and mix in honey (or sweetener) and cinnamon (if using) until well combined.
2. **Add Berries:** Gently fold in the mixed berries, reserving a few for topping if desired.
3. **Top with Flaxseeds:** Sprinkle the ground flaxseeds over the cottage cheese and berry mixture.
4. **Serve:** If desired, top with additional berries and chopped nuts or seeds for added texture and flavor. Enjoy immediately.

Nutrition Information (Per Serving)

Calories	250
Protein	20g
Carbohydrates	30g
Dietary Fiber	8g
Sugars	5g
Fat	8g
Saturated Fat	2g

"You are worthy of love."

QUICK NOTES

TIPS FOR CUSTOMIZATION

- **Add Flavor:** Mix in a splash of vanilla extract for extra flavor.
- **Fruit Options:** Use any seasonal fruits or your favorite berries for topping.
- **Nut Variations:** Substitute flaxseeds with chia seeds or hemp seeds for variety.

Why is this recipe good for PCOS?

This cottage cheese bowl is high in protein, which helps regulate blood sugar levels and promotes satiety. The fiber from berries and flaxseeds aids in digestion and can help manage weight, which is beneficial for women with PCOS. This recipe is nutritious, easy to prepare, and perfect for a satisfying breakfast or snack option.

Notes

Chapter 4.

PCOS - Friendly Lunch Recipes

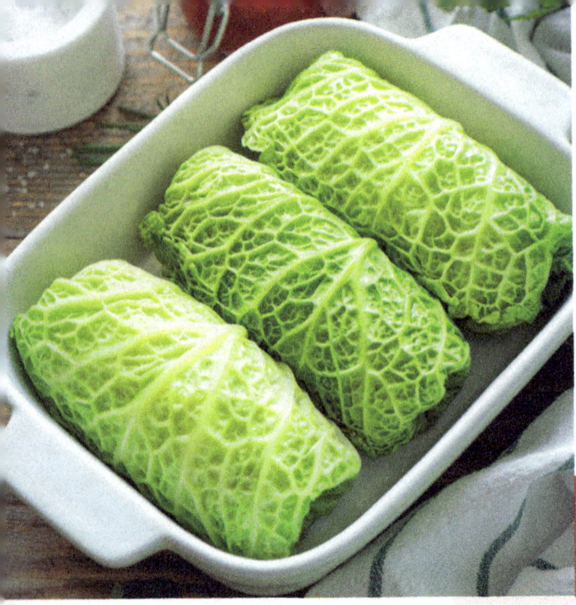

Cabbage Wraps with Spicy Chickpea Filling

SERVING SIZE
Serves 4 (2 wraps per serving)

INGREDIENTS

- 8 large cabbage leaves (green or Napa cabbage)
- 1 can (15 oz) chickpeas, drained and rinsed
- 1 small onion, diced
- 2 cloves garlic, minced
- 1 tablespoon olive oil
- 1 teaspoon cumin
- 1 teaspoon smoked paprika
- 1/2 teaspoon cayenne pepper (adjust to taste)
- Salt and pepper to taste
- 1 avocado, sliced (for serving)
- Fresh cilantro or parsley for garnish (optional)

DIRECTIONS

1. **Prepare Cabbage Leaves:** Bring a large pot of water to a boil. Carefully add the cabbage leaves and blanch for 2-3 minutes until softened. Remove and place in a bowl of ice water to stop the cooking process. Drain and set aside.
2. **Cook Filling:** In a skillet, heat olive oil over medium heat. Add diced onion and sauté until translucent, about 3-4 minutes. Stir in minced garlic and cook for another minute.
3. **Add Chickpeas and Spices:** Add the chickpeas to the skillet, along with cumin, smoked paprika, cayenne pepper, salt, and pepper. Mash the chickpeas slightly with a fork or potato masher, mixing well. Cook for about 5 minutes until heated through.
4. **Assemble Wraps:** Take a cabbage leaf and spoon a portion of the chickpea filling into the center. Fold the sides over the filling and roll up tightly. Repeat with remaining leaves and filling.
5. **Serve:** Serve the cabbage wraps with sliced avocado on the side. Garnish with fresh cilantro or parsley if desired.

Nutrition Information (Per Serving)

Calories	300
Protein	12g
Fat	15g
Carbohydrates	30g
Fiber	10g
Sugar	3g

"Your voice is important."

QUICK NOTES

TIPS FOR CUSTOMIZATION

- **Spices:** Adjust the spice level by adding more or less cayenne pepper or including other spices like curry powder or chili powder.
- **Vegetables:** Add diced bell peppers, carrots, or spinach to the chickpea filling for extra nutrition.
- **Sauce:** Drizzle with tahini or a yogurt alternative for added creaminess.

Why is this recipe good for PCOS?

- **High Fiber:** Chickpeas and cabbage are high in fiber, which helps regulate blood sugar levels and supports digestive health.
- **Plant-Based Protein:** Chickpeas provide a good source of plant-based protein, beneficial for hormone balance.
- **Low Carb:** This dish is relatively low in carbohydrates, making it suitable for those managing insulin resistance.
- **Nutrient-Dense:** The combination of vegetables and healthy fats from avocado adds vitamins, minerals, and antioxidants, promoting overall health.

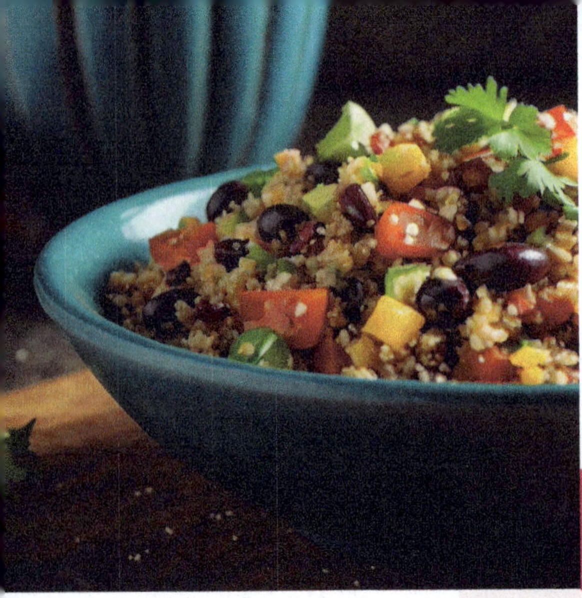

Quinoa and Black Bean Salad with Lime Dressing

SERVING SIZE
Serves 4

INGREDIENTS

- 1 cup quinoa, rinsed
- 2 cups water or vegetable broth
- 1 can (15 oz) black beans, drained and rinsed
- 1 cup corn (fresh, frozen, or canned)
- 1 bell pepper, diced (any color)
- 1 small red onion, diced
- 1/4 cup fresh cilantro, chopped
- 1/4 cup olive oil
- 1/4 cup fresh lime juice (about 2 limes)
- 1 teaspoon cumin
- Salt and pepper to taste

DIRECTIONS

1. **Cook Quinoa:** In a medium saucepan, combine quinoa and water or vegetable broth. Bring to a boil, then reduce heat to low, cover, and simmer for about 15 minutes, or until the quinoa is fluffy and the liquid is absorbed. Remove from heat and let it cool.
2. **Prepare Salad Ingredients:** In a large bowl, combine black beans, corn, diced bell pepper, red onion, and chopped cilantro.
3. **Make Dressing:** In a small bowl, whisk together olive oil, lime juice, cumin, salt, and pepper.
4. **Combine:** Once the quinoa has cooled, add it to the bowl with the vegetables. Pour the lime dressing over the salad and toss to combine.
5. **Serve:** Serve immediately or refrigerate for 30 minutes to allow the flavors to meld.

Nutrition Information (Per Serving)

Calories	320
Protein	12g
Fat	14g
Carbohydrates	42g
Fiber	10g
Sugar	3g

"Celebrate small victories."

QUICK NOTES

TIPS FOR CUSTOMIZATION

- **Vegetables:** Add other vegetables like diced cucumbers, cherry tomatoes, or avocado for extra flavor and nutrition.
- **Spice Level:** Add diced jalapeños or a pinch of cayenne pepper for a spicy kick.
- **Protein:** Include grilled chicken, shrimp, or tofu for added protein.

Why is this recipe good for PCOS?

- **High Fiber:** Quinoa and black beans are rich in fiber, which helps regulate blood sugar levels and supports digestive health.
- **Plant-Based Protein:** This salad provides a good source of plant-based protein, beneficial for hormone balance.
- **Nutrient-Dense:** The variety of vegetables adds vitamins, minerals, and antioxidants, promoting overall health.
- **Low Glycemic Index:** Quinoa and black beans have a low glycemic index, making them suitable for those managing insulin resistance.

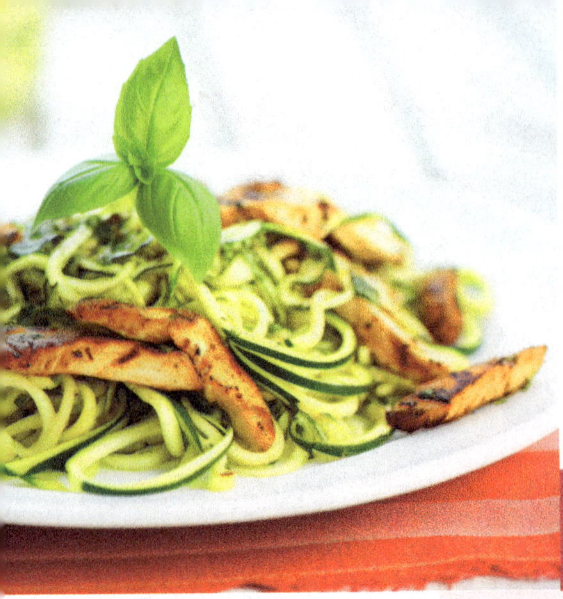

Zucchini Noodle Salad with Grilled Chicken and Avocado

SERVING SIZE
Serves 4

INGREDIENTS

- 2 medium zucchinis, spiralized into noodles
- 1 lb (450g) grilled chicken breast, sliced
- 1 avocado, diced
- 1 cup cherry tomatoes, halved
- 1/4 cup red onion, thinly sliced (optional)
- 1/4 cup fresh basil or parsley, chopped (for garnish)

For the Lemon Vinaigrette

- 1/4 cup olive oil
  2 tablespoons fresh lemon juice (about 1 lemon)
- 1 teaspoon Dijon mustard
- 1 clove garlic, minced
- Salt and pepper to taste

DIRECTIONS

1. **Prepare Zucchini Noodles:** Spiralize the zucchinis into noodles using a spiralizer. If you don't have one, you can use a vegetable peeler to create thin strips.
2. **Make Vinaigrette:** In a small bowl, whisk together olive oil, lemon juice, Dijon mustard, minced garlic, salt, and pepper until well combined.
3. **Combine Salad Ingredients:** In a large bowl, combine the spiralized zucchini, grilled chicken, diced avocado, cherry tomatoes, and red onion (if using).
4. **Dress the Salad:** Pour the lemon vinaigrette over the salad and toss gently to combine, being careful not to mash the avocado.
5. **Serve:** Garnish with fresh basil or parsley and serve immediately.

Nutrition Information (Per Serving)

Calories	320
Protein	30g
Fat	20g
Carbohydrates	12g
Fiber	6g
Sugar	3g

"You can do hard things."

QUICK NOTES

TIPS FOR CUSTOMIZATION

- **Protein:** Substitute grilled chicken with shrimp, turkey, or tofu for a different protein source.
- **Vegetables:** Add other vegetables like bell peppers, cucumbers, or spinach for extra nutrition.
- **Spice Level:** Add red pepper flakes or a dash of hot sauce to the vinaigrette for a spicy kick.

Why is this recipe good for PCOS?

- **Low Carb:** Zucchini noodles are a low-carb alternative to traditional pasta, making it suitable for those managing insulin resistance.
- **High Protein:** Grilled chicken provides lean protein, which helps stabilize blood sugar levels.
- **Healthy Fats:** Avocado adds healthy fats that can support hormone balance and satiety.
- **Nutrient-Dense:** The combination of fresh vegetables and herbs adds vitamins, minerals, and antioxidants, promoting overall health.

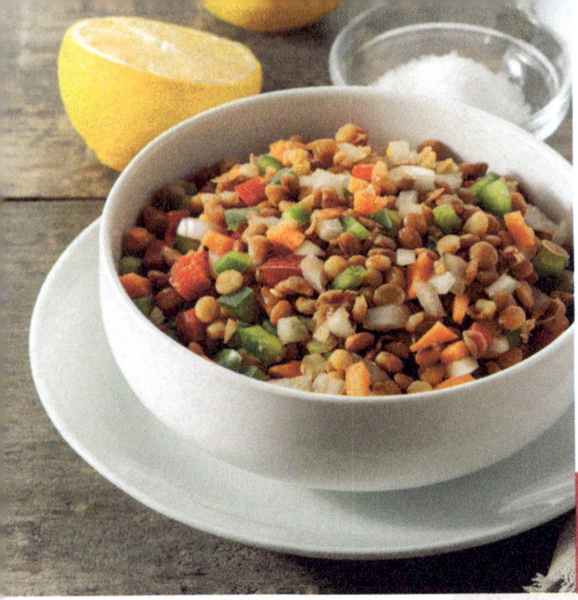

Lentil and Vegetable Stir-Fry

SERVING SIZE
Serves 4

INGREDIENTS

- 1 cup cooked lentils (green or brown)
- 2 cups mixed vegetables (e.g., bell peppers, broccoli, carrots, snap peas)
- 2 tablespoons olive oil or sesame oil
- 3 cloves garlic, minced
- 1 tablespoon ginger, minced
- 3 tablespoons soy sauce or tamari (for gluten-free)
- 1 tablespoon rice vinegar (optional)
- 1 teaspoon sesame oil (optional, for flavor)
- Salt and pepper to taste
- Cooked cauliflower rice (for serving)
- Green onions or sesame seeds for garnish (optional)

DIRECTIONS

1. **Prepare Cauliflower Rice:** If using fresh cauliflower, pulse it in a food processor until it resembles rice. Sauté in a pan with a little olive oil for about 5 minutes until tender. Alternatively, you can use pre-packaged cauliflower rice.
2. **Heat Oil:** In a large skillet or wok, heat the olive oil or sesame oil over medium-high heat.
3. **Sauté Aromatics:** Add minced garlic and ginger to the skillet, sautéing for about 1 minute until fragrant.
4. **Add Vegetables:** Stir in the mixed vegetables and cook for about 5-7 minutes until they are tender-crisp.
5. **Add Lentils**: Add the cooked lentils to the skillet, along with soy sauce or tamari, rice vinegar (if using), and sesame oil (if using). Stir well to combine and heat through for another 2-3 minutes.
6. **Serve:** Serve the lentil and vegetable stir-fry over cauliflower rice. Garnish with green onions or sesame seeds if desired.

Nutrition Information (Per Serving)

Calories	280
Protein	15g
Fat	10g
Carbohydrates	35g
Fiber	12g
Sugar	4g

"Your story is powerful."

QUICK NOTES

TIPS FOR CUSTOMIZATION

- **Vegetables:** Use any combination of vegetables you like or have on hand, such as zucchini, mushrooms, or spinach.
- **Spice Level:** Add red pepper flakes or sriracha for a spicy kick.
- **Protein:** Include tofu or tempeh for added protein if desired.

Why is this recipe good for PCOS?

- **High Fiber:** Lentils and vegetables are rich in fiber, which helps regulate blood sugar levels and supports digestive health.
- **Plant-Based Protein:** Lentils provide a good source of plant-based protein, beneficial for hormone balance.
- **Low Glycemic Index:** This dish has a low glycemic index, making it suitable for those managing insulin resistance.
- **Nutrient-Dense:** The variety of vegetables adds vitamins, minerals, and antioxidants, promoting overall health.

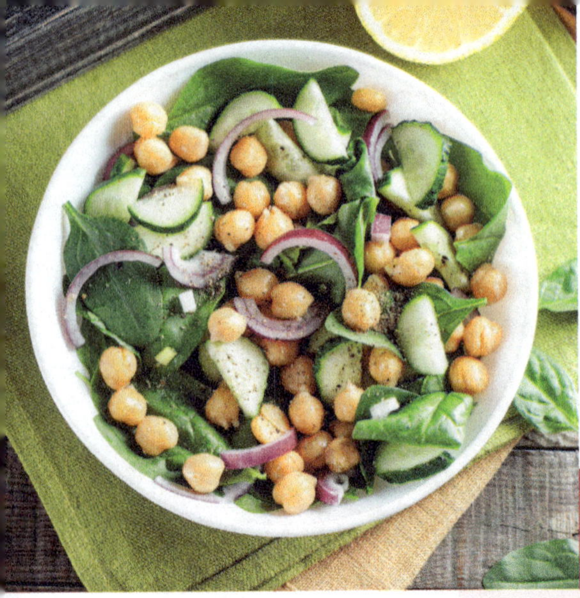

Chickpea and Spinach Salad with Tahini Dressing

SERVING SIZE
Serves 4

INGREDIENTS

- 1 can (15 oz) chickpeas, drained and rinsed
- 4 cups fresh spinach, washed and dried
- 1 cup cherry tomatoes, halved
- 1/2 cucumber, diced
- 1/4 red onion, thinly sliced
- 1/4 cup fresh parsley or cilantro, chopped (optional)
- 1/4 cup tahini
- 2 tablespoons lemon juice (about 1 lemon)
- 1 tablespoon olive oil
- 1 clove garlic, minced
  Water (to thin the dressing)
- Salt and pepper to taste

DIRECTIONS

1. **Prepare Salad Ingredients:** In a large bowl, combine chickpeas, spinach, cherry tomatoes, cucumber, red onion, and parsley or cilantro (if using).
2. **Make Tahini Dressing:** In a small bowl, whisk together tahini, lemon juice, olive oil, minced garlic, salt, and pepper. Add water a tablespoon at a time until the dressing reaches your desired consistency.
3. **Combine:** Pour the tahini dressing over the salad and toss gently to combine, ensuring all ingredients are well coated.
4. **Serve:** Serve immediately or let it sit for 10-15 minutes to allow the flavors to meld.

Nutrition Information (Per Serving)

Calories	280
Protein	10g
Fat	18g
Carbohydrates	25g
Fiber	8g
Sugar	3g

"Stay hopeful and strong."

QUICK NOTES

TIPS FOR CUSTOMIZATION

- **Vegetables:** Add other vegetables like bell peppers, carrots, or radishes for extra crunch and nutrition.
- **Protein:** Include grilled chicken, shrimp, or tofu for added protein.
- **Spice Level:** Add a pinch of cayenne pepper or red pepper flakes to the dressing for a spicy kick.

Why is this recipe good for PCOS?

- **High Fiber:** Chickpeas and spinach are rich in fiber, which helps regulate blood sugar levels and supports digestive health.
- **Plant-Based Protein:** Chickpeas provide a good source of plant-based protein, beneficial for hormone balance.
- **Healthy Fats:** Tahini and olive oil provide healthy fats that can support hormone balance and satiety.
- **Nutrient-Dense:** The combination of fresh vegetables adds vitamins, minerals, and antioxidants, promoting overall health.

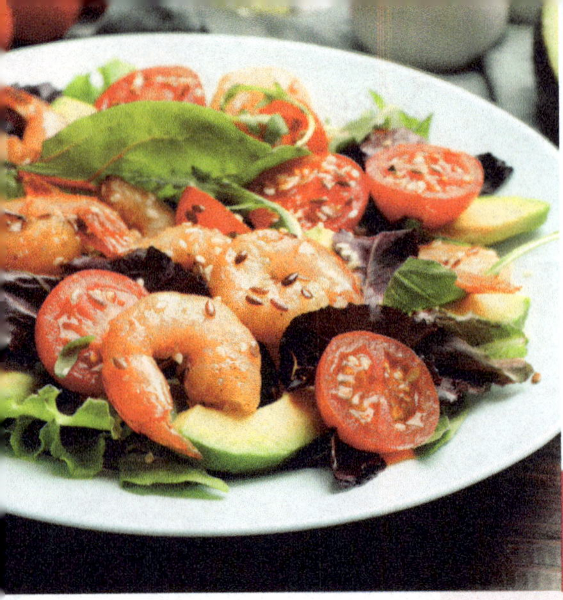

Grilled Shrimp Salad with Avocado and Citrus Dressing

SERVING SIZE
Serves 4

INGREDIENTS

- 1 lb (450g) shrimp, peeled and deveined
- 4 cups mixed greens (e.g., spinach, arugula, romaine)
- 1 avocado, diced
- 1 cup cherry tomatoes, halved
- 1/4 red onion, thinly sliced
- 1/4 cup fresh cilantro or parsley, chopped (optional)

For the Citrus Dressing

- 1/4 cup olive oil
- 2 tablespoons fresh orange juice (about 1 orange)
- 1 tablespoon fresh lime juice (about 1 lime)
- 1 teaspoon honey or maple syrup (optional)
- Salt and pepper to taste

DIRECTIONS

1. **Preheat Grill:** Preheat your grill to medium-high heat.
   Prepare Shrimp: In a bowl, toss the shrimp with a drizzle of olive oil, salt, and pepper. If desired, add minced garlic or spices for extra flavor.
2. **Grill Shrimp:** Place the shrimp on the grill and cook for about 2-3 minutes per side, or until they are pink and opaque. Remove from the grill and set aside.
3. **Make Citrus Dressing:** In a small bowl, whisk together olive oil, orange juice, lime juice, honey (if using), salt, and pepper until well combined.
4. **Assemble Salad:** In a large bowl, combine mixed greens, diced avocado, cherry tomatoes, and red onion. Add the grilled shrimp on top.
5. **Dress Salad:** Drizzle the citrus dressing over the salad and toss gently to combine.
6. **Serve:** Garnish with fresh cilantro or parsley if desired and serve immediately.

Nutrition Information (Per Serving)

Calories	320
Protein	25g
Fat	20g
Carbohydrates	15g
Fiber	6g
Sugar	3g

"You are a warrior."

QUICK NOTES

TIPS FOR CUSTOMIZATION

- **Vegetables:** Add other vegetables like bell peppers, cucumbers, or radishes for extra crunch and nutrition.
- **Protein:** Substitute shrimp with grilled chicken, tofu, or fish for a different protein source.
- **Spice Level:** Add a pinch of red pepper flakes or a dash of hot sauce to the dressing for a spicy kick.

Why is this recipe good for PCOS?

- **High Protein:** Shrimp provides lean protein, which helps stabilize blood sugar levels.
- **Healthy Fats:** Avocado and olive oil provide healthy fats that can support hormone balance and satiety.
- **Low Carb:** This salad is low in carbohydrates, making it suitable for those managing insulin resistance.
- **Nutrient-Dense:** The combination of fresh vegetables and citrus dressing adds vitamins, minerals, and antioxidants, promoting overall health.

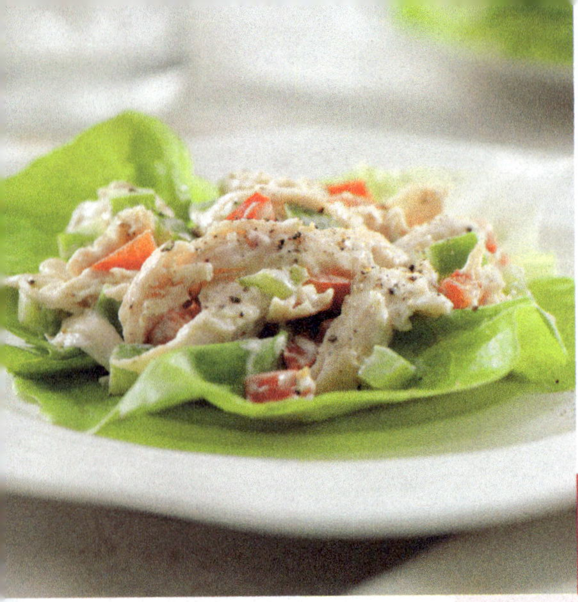

Egg Salad Lettuce Wraps

SERVING SIZE
Serves 4 (2 wraps per serving)

INGREDIENTS

- 6 large eggs
- 1 ripe avocado, mashed
- 1 tablespoon Dijon mustard
- 1 tablespoon fresh lemon juice
- 1/4 cup red onion, finely chopped
- 1/4 cup celery, finely chopped
- Salt and pepper to taste
- 8 large lettuce leaves (e.g., romaine, butter, or iceberg)
- Fresh herbs for garnish (optional, e.g., dill or parsley)

DIRECTIONS

1. **Boil Eggs:** Place the eggs in a pot and cover with water. Bring to a boil, then reduce heat and simmer for 9-12 minutes. Remove from heat and transfer the eggs to an ice bath to cool. Once cooled, peel the eggs and chop them.
2. **Make Egg Salad:** In a mixing bowl, combine the chopped eggs, mashed avocado, Dijon mustard, lemon juice, red onion, celery, salt, and pepper. Mix until well combined and creamy.
3. **Prepare Lettuce Wraps:** Carefully separate the lettuce leaves and lay them flat on a serving platter.
4. **Assemble Wraps:** Spoon the egg salad mixture into the center of each lettuce leaf.
5. **Serve:** Garnish with fresh herbs if desired and serve immediately.

Nutrition Information (Per Serving)

Calories	250
Protein	12g
Fat	20g
Carbohydrates	10g
Fiber	5g
Sugar	1g

"Trust your journey."

QUICK NOTES

TIPS FOR CUSTOMIZATION

- **Add-ins:** Include diced bell peppers, pickles, or capers for extra flavor and crunch.
- **Spices:** Add a pinch of paprika or cayenne pepper for a spicy kick.
- **Herbs:** Experiment with different herbs like chives, dill, or cilantro for varied flavors.

Why is this recipe good for PCOS?

- **High Protein:** Eggs provide high-quality protein, which helps stabilize blood sugar levels.
- **Healthy Fats:** Avocado adds healthy fats that can support hormone balance and satiety.
- **Low Carb:** This dish is low in carbohydrates, making it suitable for those managing insulin resistance.
- **Nutrient-Dense:** The combination of eggs and fresh vegetables adds vitamins, minerals, and antioxidants, promoting overall health.

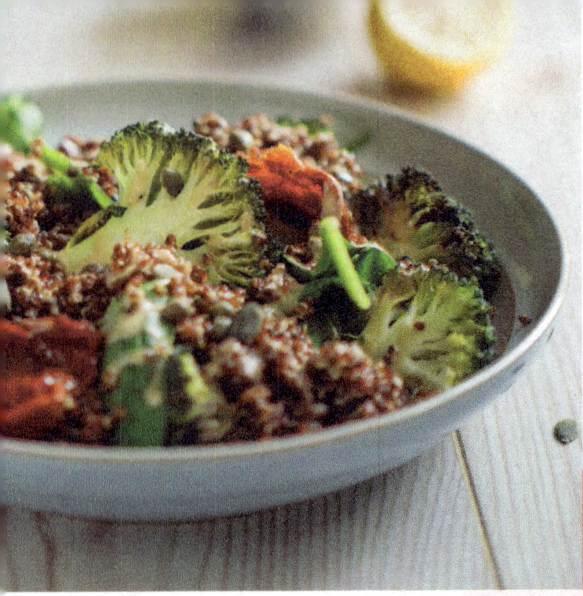

Roasted Vegetable and Quinoa Bowl

SERVING SIZE
Serves 4

INGREDIENTS

- 1 cup quinoa, rinsed
- 2 cups water or vegetable broth
- 2 cups seasonal vegetables (e.g., bell peppers, zucchini, carrots, broccoli), chopped
- 2 tablespoons olive oil
- Salt and pepper to taste
- 1 teaspoon garlic powder (optional)
- 1 teaspoon smoked paprika (optional)

For the Tahini Dressing

- 1/4 cup tahini
- 2 tablespoons lemon juice (about 1 lemon)
- 1 tablespoon maple syrup or honey (optional)
- 2-3 tablespoons water (to thin the dressing)
- Salt to taste

DIRECTIONS

1. **Preheat Oven:** Preheat your oven to 400°F (200°C).
2. **Cook Quinoa:** In a medium saucepan, combine quinoa and water or vegetable broth. Bring to a boil, then reduce heat to low, cover, and simmer for about 15 minutes, or until the quinoa is fluffy and the liquid is absorbed. Remove from heat and let it cool.
3. **Prepare Vegetables:** On a baking sheet, toss the chopped vegetables with olive oil, salt, pepper, garlic powder, and smoked paprika. Spread them out in a single layer.
4. **Roast Vegetables:** Roast in the preheated oven for 20-25 minutes, or until the vegetables are tender and slightly caramelized, stirring halfway through.
5. **Make Tahini Dressing:** In a small bowl, whisk together tahini, lemon juice, maple syrup (if using), water, and salt until smooth. Adjust the consistency by adding more water if needed.
6. **Assemble Bowl:** In a serving bowl, layer cooked quinoa and top with roasted vegetables. Drizzle with tahini dressing.
7. **Serve:** Serve warm, garnished with fresh herbs if desired.

Nutrition Information (Per Serving)

Calories	350
Protein	12g
Fat	18g
Carbohydrates	40g
Fiber	8g
Sugar	3g

"You define your path."

QUICK NOTES

TIPS FOR CUSTOMIZATION

- **Vegetables:** Use any seasonal vegetables you like or have on hand, such as sweet potatoes, Brussels sprouts, or asparagus.
- **Grains:** Substitute quinoa with brown rice, farro, or bulgur for variety.
- **Add Protein:** Include grilled chicken, chickpeas, or tofu for added protein.

Why is this recipe good for PCOS?

- **High Fiber:** Quinoa and vegetables are rich in fiber, which helps regulate blood sugar levels and supports digestive health.
- **Plant-Based Protein:** Quinoa provides a good source of plant-based protein, beneficial for hormone balance.
- **Nutrient-Dense:** The variety of vegetables adds vitamins, minerals, and antioxidants, promoting overall health.
- **Healthy Fats:** Tahini provides healthy fats that can support hormone balance and satiety.

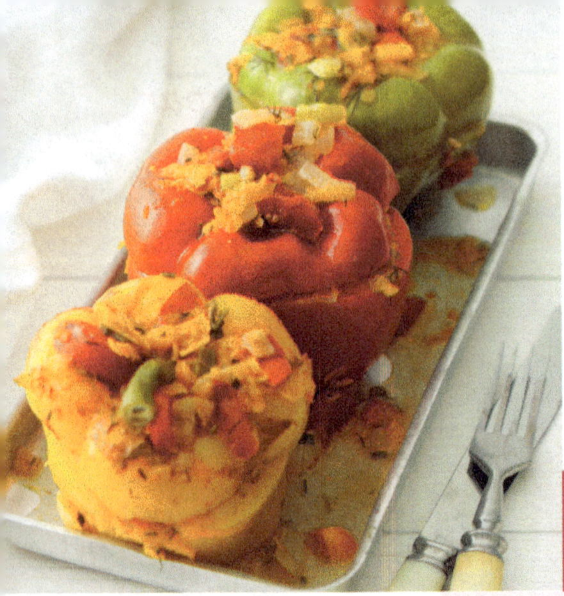

Stuffed Bell Peppers with Turkey and Cauliflower Rice

SERVING SIZE
Serves 4

INGREDIENTS

- 4 large bell peppers (any color)
- 1 lb (450g) ground turkey
- 1 cup cauliflower rice (fresh or frozen)
- 1 can (15 oz) diced tomatoes (no added sugar)
- 1 small onion, diced
- 2 cloves garlic, minced
- 1 teaspoon Italian seasoning
- 1 teaspoon paprika
- Salt and pepper to taste
- 1 tablespoon olive oil
- Fresh parsley or basil for garnish (optional)

DIRECTIONS

1. **Preheat Oven:** Preheat your oven to 375°F (190°C).
2. **Prepare Peppers:** Cut the tops off the bell peppers and remove the seeds. Place them upright in a baking dish.
3. **Cook Filling:** In a large skillet, heat olive oil over medium heat. Add diced onion and garlic, sautéing until softened. Add ground turkey and cook until browned. Stir in cauliflower rice, diced tomatoes, Italian seasoning, paprika, salt, and pepper. Cook for an additional 5 minutes until heated through.
4. **Stuff Peppers:** Spoon the filling into each bell pepper, packing it down gently.
5. **Bake:** Cover the baking dish with foil and bake for 25-30 minutes. Remove the foil and bake for an additional 10 minutes, until the peppers are tender.
6. **Serve:** Garnish with fresh parsley or basil if desired, and serve hot.

Nutrition Information (Per Serving)

Calories	280
Protein	25g
Fat	10g
Carbohydrates	20g
Fiber	5g
Sugar	5g

"Your feelings are valid."

QUICK NOTES

TIPS FOR CUSTOMIZATION

- **Protein:** Substitute ground turkey with ground chicken, beef, or a plant-based protein for a vegetarian option.
- **Vegetables:** Add chopped spinach, mushrooms, or zucchini to the filling for extra nutrients.
- **Spices:** Experiment with different spices like cumin or chili powder for added flavor.

Why is this recipe good for PCOS?

- **High Protein:** The ground turkey provides lean protein, which helps stabilize blood sugar levels.
- **Low Carb:** Using cauliflower rice keeps the dish low in carbohydrates, beneficial for insulin sensitivity.
- **Nutrient-Dense:** Bell peppers are rich in vitamins A and C, antioxidants that support overall health.
- **Fiber-Rich:** The combination of vegetables and protein helps promote satiety and digestive health.

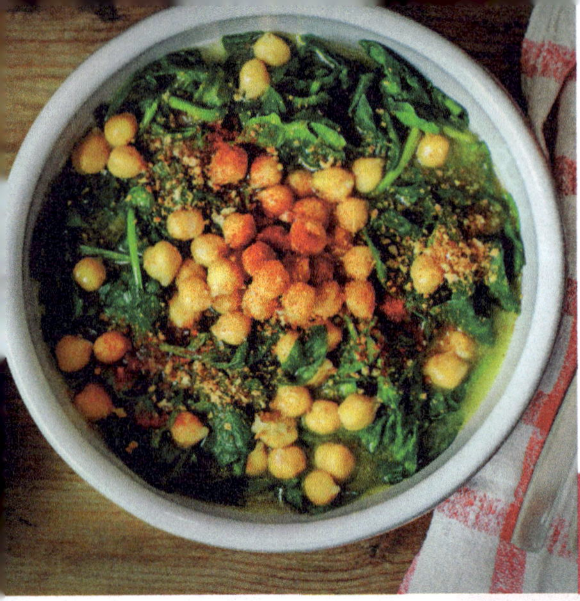

Chickpea and Spinach Stew

SERVING SIZE
Serves 4

INGREDIENTS

- 1 can (15 oz) chickpeas, drained and rinsed
- 4 cups fresh spinach (or 1 can of spinach, drained)
- 1 can (14 oz) diced tomatoes (no added sugar)
- 1 small onion, diced
- 3 cloves garlic, minced
- 1 teaspoon ground cumin
- 1 teaspoon smoked paprika
- 1/2 teaspoon turmeric
- 1/2 teaspoon red pepper flakes (optional, for heat)
- 2 tablespoons olive oil
- 2 cups vegetable broth or water
- Salt and pepper to taste
- Fresh cilantro or parsley for garnish (optional)

DIRECTIONS

1. **Heat Oil:** In a large pot, heat olive oil over medium heat. Add diced onion and sauté until translucent, about 5 minutes.
2. **Add Garlic and Spices:** Stir in minced garlic, cumin, smoked paprika, turmeric, and red pepper flakes (if using). Cook for another minute until fragrant.
3. **Add Tomatoes and Broth:** Pour in the diced tomatoes and vegetable broth. Bring to a simmer.
4. **Add Chickpeas:** Stir in the chickpeas and season with salt and pepper. Simmer for about 10-15 minutes, allowing the flavors to meld.
5. **Add Spinach:** Stir in the fresh spinach and cook for an additional 2-3 minutes until wilted.
6. **Serve:** Ladle the stew into bowls and garnish with fresh cilantro or parsley if desired.

Nutrition Information (Per Serving)

Calories	220
Protein	10g
Fat	8g
Carbohydrates	30g
Fiber	10g
Sugar	4g

"Keep pushing forward."

QUICK NOTES

TIPS FOR CUSTOMIZATION

- **Vegetables:** Add other vegetables like carrots, bell peppers, or zucchini for extra nutrition.
- **Spices:** Adjust the spices to your taste; add curry powder or coriander for different flavor profiles.
- **Protein:** Include cooked chicken or tofu for added protein if desired.

Why is this recipe good for PCOS?

- **High Fiber:** Chickpeas and spinach are rich in fiber, which helps regulate blood sugar levels and supports digestive health.
- **Plant-Based Protein:** Chickpeas provide a good source of plant-based protein, beneficial for hormone balance.
- **Nutrient-Dense:** The combination of vegetables and spices adds vitamins, minerals, and antioxidants, promoting overall health.
- **Low Glycemic Index:** This stew has a low glycemic index, making it suitable for those managing insulin resistance.

Notes

5.

Chapter

PCOS - Friendly

Dinner Recipes

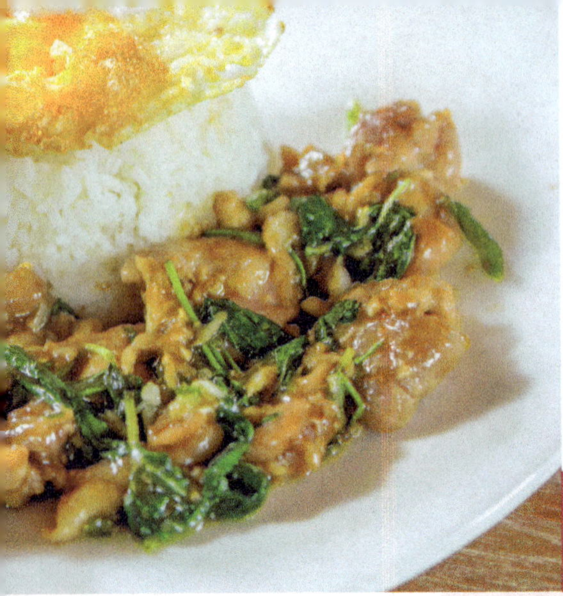

Thai Basil Chicken

SERVING SIZE
Serves 4

INGREDIENTS

- 1 lb (450g) ground chicken
- 1 cup fresh Thai basil leaves
- 2 tablespoons coconut oil (or olive oil)
- 4 cloves garlic, minced
- 2-3 Thai bird's eye chilies, chopped (adjust to taste)
- 2 tablespoons coconut aminos (or soy sauce)
- 1 tablespoon fish sauce (optional)
- 1 tablespoon lime juice
  1 bell pepper, sliced (optional)
- 1 small onion, sliced (optional)
- Salt and pepper to taste

DIRECTIONS

1. **Heat Oil:** In a large skillet or wok, heat the coconut oil over medium-high heat.
2. **Sauté Aromatics:** Add minced garlic and chopped chilies. Sauté for about 30 seconds until fragrant.
3. **Cook Chicken:** Add the ground chicken to the skillet. Cook until browned and cooked through, breaking it apart with a spatula.
4. **Add Vegetables:** If using, add sliced bell pepper and onion. Stir-fry for 2-3 minutes until vegetables are tender.
5. **Season:** Stir in coconut aminos, fish sauce (if using), lime juice, salt, and pepper. Mix well.
6. **Add Basil:** Remove from heat and fold in the fresh Thai basil leaves until wilted.
7. **Serve:** Serve hot, optionally over cauliflower rice or zucchini noodles.

Nutrition Information (Per Serving)

Calories	250
Protein	25g
Fat	15g
Carbohydrates	5g
Fiber	1g
Sugar	1g

"You are capable of change."

QUICK NOTES

TIPS FOR CUSTOMIZATION

- **Protein:** Substitute ground chicken with ground turkey, beef, or tofu for a vegetarian option.
- **Vegetables:** Add other vegetables like snap peas, carrots, or broccoli for more nutrition.
- **Spice Level:** Adjust the number of chilies based on your spice preference.

Why is this recipe good for PCOS?

- **High Protein:** The ground chicken provides lean protein, which helps in managing blood sugar levels.
- **Low Carb:** This dish is low in carbohydrates, making it suitable for those managing insulin resistance.
- **Nutrient-Dense:** The addition of fresh basil and vegetables adds vitamins and antioxidants, supporting overall health.
- **Healthy Fats:** Coconut oil provides healthy fats that can help with hormone balance.

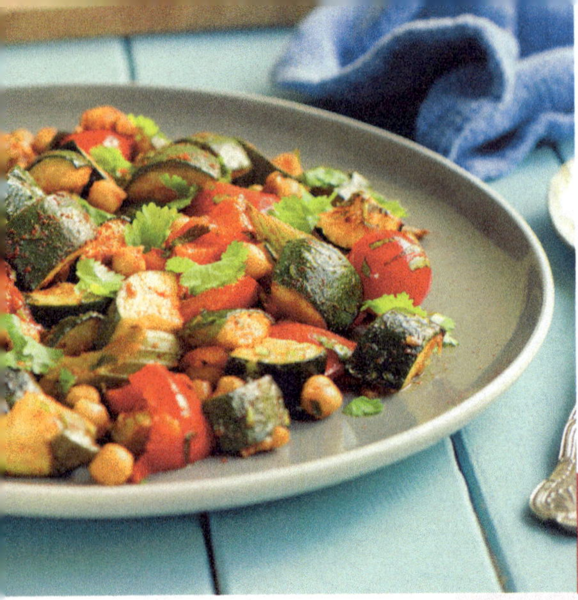

Roasted Vegetable and Chickpea Bowl

SERVING SIZE
Serves 4

INGREDIENTS

- 1 can (15 oz) chickpeas, drained and rinsed
- 2 cups mixed vegetables (e.g., bell peppers, zucchini, carrots, and red onion)
- 2 tablespoons olive oil
- 1 teaspoon garlic powder
- 1 teaspoon smoked paprika
- 1 teaspoon cumin
- Salt and pepper to taste
- 2 cups fresh spinach or kale
- 1 avocado, sliced (for topping)
- Lemon wedges (for serving)

DIRECTIONS

1. **Preheat Oven:** Preheat your oven to 400°F (200°C).
2. **Prepare Vegetables:** In a large bowl, combine the mixed vegetables and chickpeas. Drizzle with olive oil and sprinkle with garlic powder, smoked paprika, cumin, salt, and pepper. Toss to coat evenly.
3. **Roast:** Spread the mixture on a baking sheet in a single layer. Roast in the preheated oven for 25-30 minutes, or until the vegetables are tender and slightly caramelized.
4. **Serve:** In a bowl, layer fresh spinach or kale, then top with the roasted vegetable and chickpea mixture. Add sliced avocado on top and serve with lemon wedges.

Nutrition Information (Per Serving)

Calories	350
Protein	12g
Fat	15g
Carbohydrates	45g
Fiber	12g
Sugar	5g

"Nourish your body with love."

QUICK NOTES

TIPS FOR CUSTOMIZATION

- **Vegetables:** Use any seasonal vegetables you have on hand, such as sweet potatoes, Brussels sprouts, or broccoli.
- **Grains:** Add cooked quinoa or brown rice for extra fiber and protein.
- **Spices:** Experiment with different spices like curry powder or Italian herbs for varied flavors.

Why is this recipe good for PCOS?

- **High Fiber:** Chickpeas and vegetables provide fiber, which helps regulate blood sugar levels and supports digestive health.
- **Nutrient-Dense:** Packed with vitamins, minerals, and antioxidants from a variety of vegetables.
- **Plant-Based Protein:** Chickpeas offer a good source of plant-based protein, which is beneficial for hormone balance.
- **Healthy Fats:** Avocado adds healthy fats that can help with satiety and overall health.

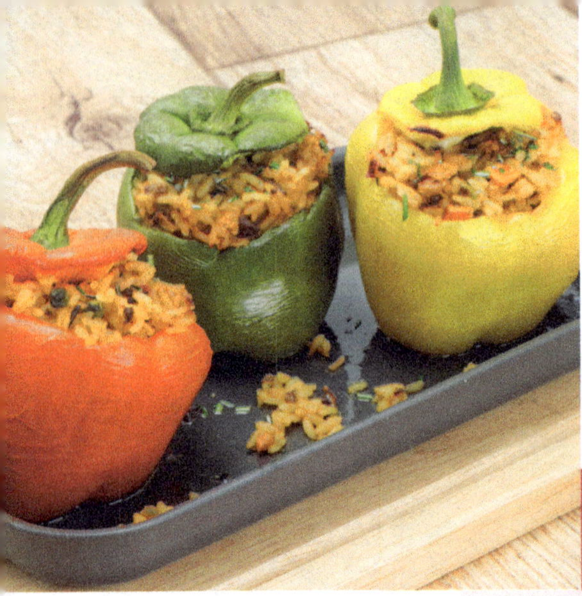

Stuffed Bell Peppers

SERVING SIZE
Serves 4

INGREDIENTS

- 4 large bell peppers (any color)
- 1 lb (450g) ground turkey or beef
- 1 cup cauliflower rice (fresh or frozen)
- 1 can (15 oz) diced tomatoes (no added sugar)
- 1 small onion, diced
- 2 cloves garlic, minced
- 1 teaspoon Italian seasoning
- 1 teaspoon paprika
- Salt and pepper to taste
- 1 tablespoon olive oil
- Fresh parsley or basil for garnish (optional)

DIRECTIONS

1. **Preheat Oven:** Preheat your oven to 375°F (190°C).
2. **Prepare Peppers:** Cut the tops off the bell peppers and remove the seeds. Place them upright in a baking dish.
3. **Cook Filling:** In a large skillet, heat olive oil over medium heat. Add diced onion and garlic, sautéing until softened. Add ground turkey or beef, cooking until browned. Stir in cauliflower rice, diced tomatoes, Italian seasoning, paprika, salt, and pepper. Cook for an additional 5 minutes until heated through.
4. **Stuff Peppers:** Spoon the filling into each bell pepper, packing it down gently.
5. **Bake:** Cover the baking dish with foil and bake for 25-30 minutes. Remove the foil and bake for an additional 10 minutes, until the peppers are tender.
6. **Serve:** Garnish with fresh parsley or basil if desired, and serve hot.

Nutrition Information (Per Serving)

Calories	280
Protein	25g
Fat	10g
Carbohydrates	20g
Fiber	5g
Sugar	5g

"You are beautiful just as you are."

QUICK NOTES

TIPS FOR CUSTOMIZATION

- **Protein:** Substitute ground turkey with ground chicken, beef, or a plant-based protein for a vegetarian option.
- **Vegetables:** Add chopped spinach, mushrooms, or zucchini to the filling for extra nutrients.
- **Spices:** Experiment with different spices like cumin or chili powder for added flavor.

Why is this recipe good for PCOS?

- **High Protein:** The ground turkey or beef provides lean protein, which helps stabilize blood sugar levels.
- **Low Carb:** Using cauliflower rice keeps the dish low in carbohydrates, beneficial for insulin sensitivity.
- **Nutrient-Dense:** Bell peppers are rich in vitamins A and C, antioxidants that support overall health.
- **Fiber-Rich:** The combination of vegetables and protein helps promote satiety and digestive health.

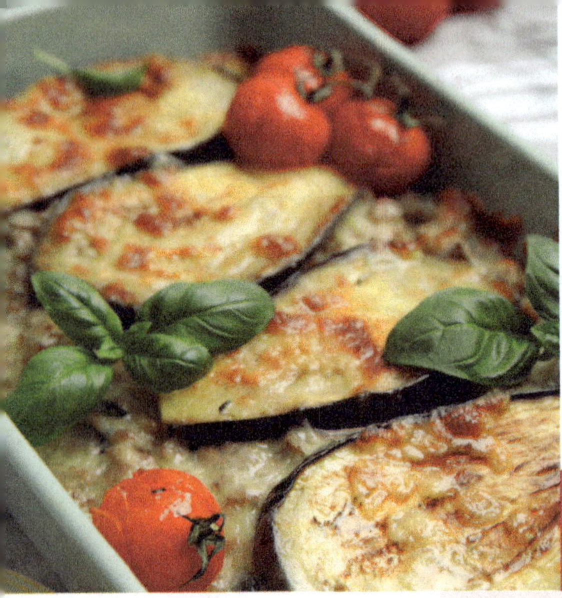

Eggplant Lasagna

SERVING SIZE
Serves 6

INGREDIENTS

- 2 large eggplants, sliced into
- 1/4-inch thick rounds
- 1 lb (450g) ground turkey or beef
- 2 cups marinara sauce (sugar-free)
- 1 small onion, diced
- 3 cloves garlic, minced
- 1 teaspoon Italian seasoning
- 1 teaspoon salt
- 1/2 teaspoon black pepper
- 1 cup fresh spinach (optional)
- 1/2 cup nutritional yeast (for a cheesy flavor, optional)
- Olive oil for brushing

DIRECTIONS

1. **Preheat Oven:** Preheat your oven to 375°F (190°C).
2. **Prepare Eggplant:** Lay the eggplant slices on a baking sheet. Brush both sides lightly with olive oil and sprinkle with salt. Bake for 20 minutes, flipping halfway through, until slightly softened.
3. **Cook Filling:** In a large skillet, heat a little olive oil over medium heat. Add diced onion and garlic, sautéing until softened. Add ground turkey or beef, cooking until browned. Stir in marinara sauce, Italian seasoning, salt, and pepper. If using, add fresh spinach and cook until wilted.
4. **Layer Lasagna:** In a baking dish, spread a thin layer of the meat sauce on the bottom. Layer with eggplant slices, followed by more meat sauce. Repeat layers until all ingredients are used, finishing with a layer of meat sauce on top. Sprinkle nutritional yeast on top if desired.
5. **Bake:** Cover the dish with foil and bake for 30 minutes. Remove the foil and bake for an additional 15 minutes until bubbly and golden.
6. **Serve:** Let it cool for a few minutes before slicing. Serve warm.

Nutrition Information (Per Serving)

Calories	280
Protein	25g
Fat	12g
Carbohydrates	18g
Fiber	6g
Sugar	5g

"Focus on progress, not perfection."

QUICK NOTES

TIPS FOR CUSTOMIZATION

- **Vegetables:** Add layers of zucchini, mushrooms, or bell peppers for extra nutrition.
- **Cheese:** For a dairy option, you can add ricotta or mozzarella cheese between the layers.
- **Spices:** Adjust the seasoning with red pepper flakes for a spicy kick.

Why is this recipe good for PCOS?

- **Low Carb:** Using eggplant instead of pasta keeps the dish low in carbohydrates, which is beneficial for insulin sensitivity.
- **High Protein:** The ground turkey or beef provides lean protein, helping to stabilize blood sugar levels.
- **Nutrient-Dense:** Eggplants are rich in antioxidants and fiber, supporting overall health.
- **Customizable:** This recipe can be easily adapted to include a variety of vegetables, enhancing its nutritional profile.

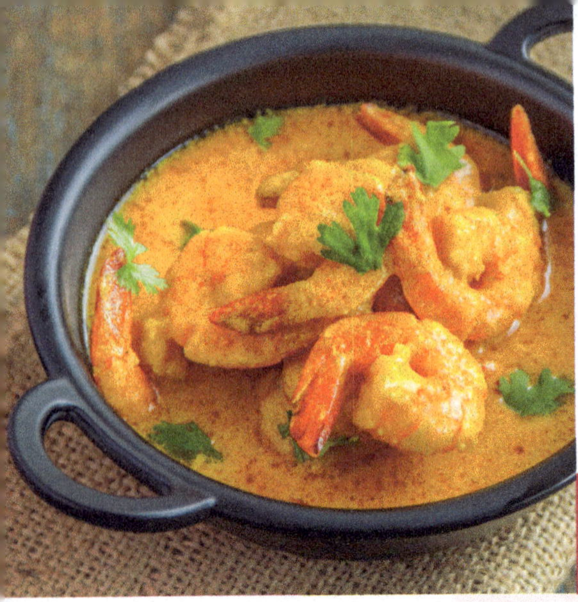

Coconut Curry Shrimp

SERVING SIZE
Serves 4

INGREDIENTS

- 1 lb (450g) shrimp, peeled and deveined
- 1 can (13.5 oz) coconut milk
- 2 tablespoons red curry paste (adjust to taste)
- 1 tablespoon olive oil or coconut oil
- 1 bell pepper, sliced
- 1 cup snap peas or green beans
- 2 cloves garlic, minced
- 1 tablespoon ginger, minced
- 1 tablespoon lime juice
- Fresh cilantro for garnish (optional)
- Salt to taste

DIRECTIONS

1. **Heat Oil:** In a large skillet, heat the olive oil or coconut oil over medium heat.
2. **Sauté Aromatics:** Add minced garlic and ginger, sautéing for about 1 minute until fragrant.
3. **Add Vegetables:** Stir in the sliced bell pepper and snap peas or green beans. Cook for 3-4 minutes until slightly tender.
4. **Add Curry Paste:** Stir in the red curry paste, mixing well with the vegetables.
5. **Add Coconut Milk:** Pour in the coconut milk and bring to a simmer. Cook for about 5 minutes, allowing the flavors to meld.
6. **Cook Shrimp:** Add the shrimp to the skillet and cook for 3-5 minutes, or until the shrimp are pink and cooked through.
7. **Finish:** Stir in lime juice and season with salt to taste. Remove from heat.
8. **Serve:** Garnish with fresh cilantro if desired and serve hot, optionally over cauliflower rice or quinoa.

Nutrition Information (Per Serving)

Calories	320
Protein	25g
Fat	20g
Carbohydrates	10g
Fiber	3g
Sugar	3g

"Your dreams are within reach."

QUICK NOTES

TIPS FOR CUSTOMIZATION

- **Vegetables:** Feel free to add other vegetables like zucchini, spinach, or carrots for added nutrition.
- **Spice Level:** Adjust the amount of red curry paste based on your spice preference.
- **Protein:** Substitute shrimp with chicken, tofu, or chickpeas for a different protein source.

Why is this recipe good for PCOS?

- **High Protein:** Shrimp provides lean protein, which helps stabilize blood sugar levels.
- **Healthy Fats:** Coconut milk contains healthy fats that can support hormone balance.
- **Low Carb:** This dish is low in carbohydrates, making it suitable for those managing insulin resistance.
- **Nutrient-Dense:** The addition of vegetables adds vitamins, minerals, and antioxidants, supporting overall health.

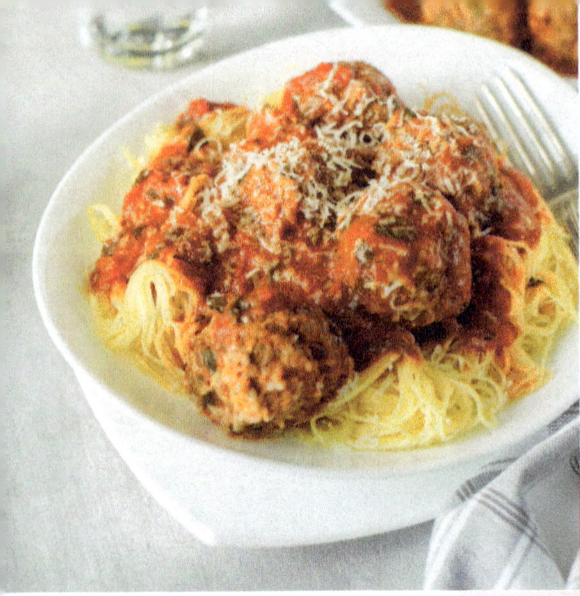

Spaghetti Squash with Meatballs

SERVING SIZE
Serves 4

INGREDIENTS

- 1 medium spaghetti squash
- 1 lb (450g) ground turkey or beef
- 1/2 cup almond flour (or gluten-free breadcrumbs)
- 1 large egg
- 2 cloves garlic, minced
- 1 teaspoon Italian seasoning
- 1 teaspoon salt
- 1/2 teaspoon black pepper
- 2 cups marinara sauce (sugar-free)
- Olive oil for drizzling
- Fresh basil or parsley for garnish (optional)

DIRECTIONS

1. **Preheat Oven:** Preheat your oven to 400°F (200°C).
2. **Prepare Spaghetti Squash:** Cut the spaghetti squash in half lengthwise and scoop out the seeds. Drizzle the inside with olive oil and sprinkle with salt and pepper. Place cut-side down on a baking sheet and roast for 30-40 minutes, or until tender.
3. **Make Meatballs:** In a large bowl, combine ground turkey or beef, almond flour, egg, minced garlic, Italian seasoning, salt, and pepper. Mix until well combined. Form into meatballs (about 1-2 inches in diameter).
4. **Cook Meatballs:** In a skillet, heat a little olive oil over medium heat. Add the meatballs and cook until browned on all sides, about 8-10 minutes. You can also bake them in the oven for about 20 minutes if preferred.
5. **Add Sauce:** Pour marinara sauce over the meatballs in the skillet and simmer for 5-10 minutes until heated through.
6. **Prepare Squash:** Once the spaghetti squash is done, use a fork to scrape the flesh into spaghetti-like strands.
7. **Serve:** Plate the spaghetti squash and top with meatballs and marinara sauce. Garnish with fresh basil or parsley if desired.

Nutrition Information (Per Serving)

Calories	320
Protein	30g
Fat	15g
Carbohydrates	18g
Fiber	5g
Sugar	5g

"You are more than your diagnosis."

QUICK NOTES

TIPS FOR CUSTOMIZATION

- **Meat Options:** Substitute ground turkey with ground chicken, beef, or a plant-based protein for a vegetarian option.
- **Sauce:** Use homemade marinara sauce for a fresher taste or add spices to enhance flavor.
- **Vegetables:** Add sautéed spinach or zucchini to the sauce for extra nutrients.

Why is this recipe good for PCOS?

- **Low Carb:** Spaghetti squash is a low-carb alternative to traditional pasta, making it suitable for those managing insulin resistance.
- **High Protein:** The meatballs provide lean protein, which helps stabilize blood sugar levels.
- **Nutrient-Dense:** This dish is rich in vitamins and minerals from the squash and any added vegetables.
- **Customizable:** Easily adaptable to include a variety of vegetables and protein sources, enhancing its nutritional profile.

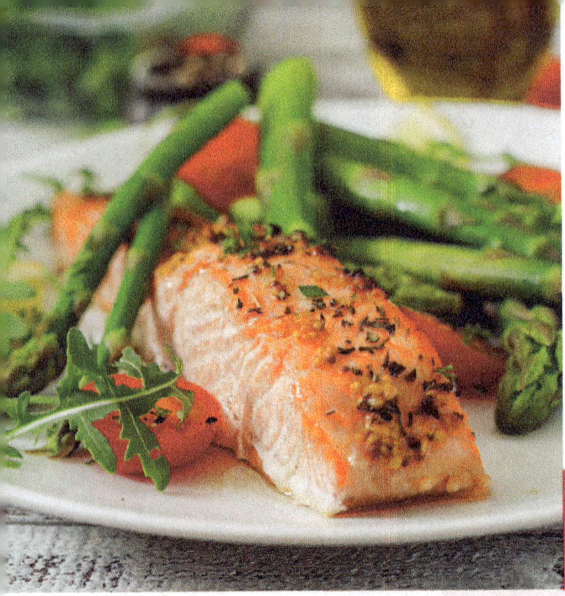

Grilled Salmon with Asparagus

SERVING SIZE
Serves 4

INGREDIENTS

- 4 salmon fillets (about 6 oz each)
- 1 lb (450g) asparagus, trimmed
- 2 tablespoons olive oil
- 2 tablespoons lemon juice
- 2 cloves garlic, minced
- 1 teaspoon dried oregano
- Salt and pepper to taste
- Lemon wedges for serving (optional)

DIRECTIONS

1. **Preheat Grill:** Preheat your grill to medium-high heat.
2. **Prepare Marinade:** In a small bowl, whisk together olive oil, lemon juice, minced garlic, oregano, salt, and pepper.
3. **Marinate Salmon:** Brush the salmon fillets with half of the marinade. Let them sit for about 10-15 minutes to absorb the flavors.
4. **Grill Asparagus:** Toss the asparagus with the remaining marinade. Place the asparagus on the grill and cook for about 5-7 minutes, turning occasionally, until tender and slightly charred.
5. **Grill Salmon:** Place the salmon fillets skin-side down on the grill. Cook for about 4-6 minutes per side, depending on thickness, until the salmon is cooked through and flakes easily with a fork.
6. **Serve:** Remove from the grill and serve hot with lemon wedges on the side.

Nutrition Information (Per Serving)

Calories	350
Protein	34g
Fat	22g
Carbohydrates	6g
Fiber	3g
Sugar	2g

"Find joy in the journey."

QUICK NOTES

TIPS FOR CUSTOMIZATION

- **Vegetables:** Substitute asparagus with other vegetables like zucchini, bell peppers, or broccoli for grilling.
- **Seasoning:** Experiment with different herbs and spices, such as dill or paprika, for varied flavors.
- **Cooking Method:** If you don't have a grill, you can also bake the salmon and asparagus in the oven at 400ºF (200ºC) for about 15-20 minutes.

Why is this recipe good for PCOS?

- **High in Omega-3s:** Salmon is rich in omega-3 fatty acids, which can help reduce inflammation and support hormone balance.
- **Low Carb:** This dish is low in carbohydrates, making it suitable for those managing insulin resistance.
- **Nutrient-Dense:** Asparagus is high in vitamins and minerals, providing antioxidants that support overall health.
- **Lean Protein:** The salmon provides high-quality protein, which helps stabilize blood sugar levels.

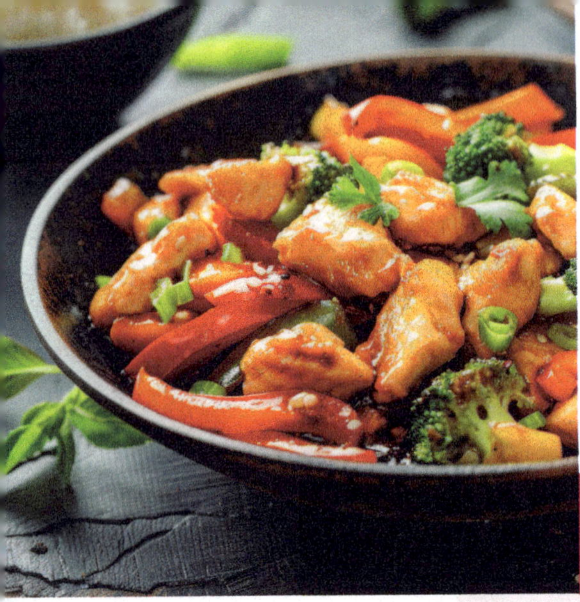

Chicken Stir-Fry

SERVING SIZE
Serves 4

INGREDIENTS

- 1 lb (450g) chicken breast, sliced into thin strips
- 2 tablespoons olive oil or sesame oil
- 2 cups mixed vegetables (e.g., bell peppers, broccoli, snap peas, carrots)
- 3 cloves garlic, minced
- 1 tablespoon ginger, minced
- 3 tablespoons coconut aminos (or soy sauce)
- 1 tablespoon rice vinegar (optional
- 1 teaspoon cornstarch (optional, for thickening)
- Salt and pepper to taste
- Cooked cauliflower rice or quinoa (for serving)

DIRECTIONS

1. **Heat Oil:** In a large skillet or wok, heat the olive oil or sesame oil over medium-high heat.
2. **Cook Chicken:** Add the sliced chicken breast to the skillet. Season with salt and pepper. Cook for about 5-7 minutes, stirring frequently, until the chicken is cooked through and no longer pink.
3. **Add Aromatics:** Stir in the minced garlic and ginger, cooking for an additional 1-2 minutes until fragrant.
4. **Add Vegetables:** Add the mixed vegetables to the skillet. Stir-fry for about 3-5 minutes until the vegetables are tender-crisp.
5. **Add Sauce:** In a small bowl, mix coconut aminos, rice vinegar, and cornstarch (if using). Pour the sauce over the chicken and vegetables, stirring to coat evenly. Cook for another 2-3 minutes until the sauce thickens slightly.
6. **Serve:** Serve hot over cauliflower rice or quinoa.

Nutrition Information (Per Serving)

Calories	300
Protein	30g
Fat	15g
Carbohydrates	10g
Fiber	3g
Sugar	4g

"You are a force of nature."

QUICK NOTES

TIPS FOR CUSTOMIZATION

- **Vegetables:** Use any combination of vegetables you like or have on hand, such as zucchini, mushrooms, or bok choy.
- **Protein:** Substitute chicken with shrimp, beef, or tofu for a different protein source.
- **Spice Level:** Add red pepper flakes or sriracha for a spicy kick.

Why is this recipe good for PCOS?

- **High Protein:** Chicken provides lean protein, which helps stabilize blood sugar levels.
- **Low Carb:** This dish is low in carbohydrates, making it suitable for those managing insulin resistance.
- **Nutrient-Dense:** The variety of vegetables adds vitamins, minerals, and antioxidants, supporting overall health.
- **Quick and Easy:** This stir-fry is quick to prepare, making it a convenient option for busy weeknights.

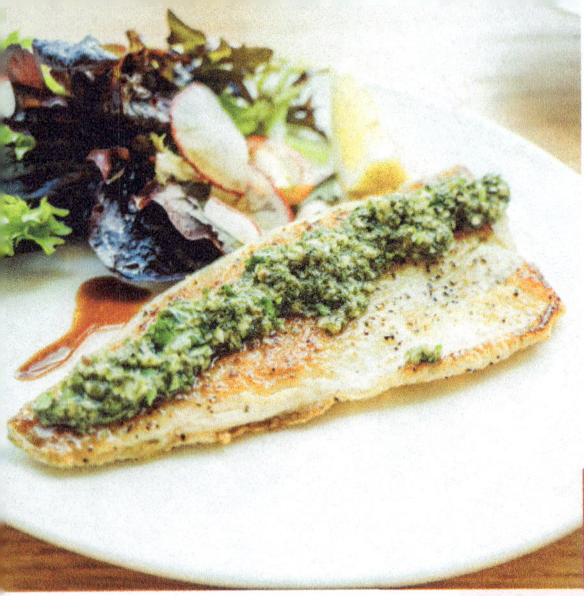

Baked Herb-Crusted Cod

SERVING SIZE
Serves 4

INGREDIENTS

- 4 cod fillets (about 6 oz each)
- 1 cup almond flour (or gluten-free breadcrumbs)
- 2 tablespoons fresh parsley, chopped
- 1 tablespoon fresh dill, chopped (or 1 teaspoon dried dill)
- 1 tablespoon fresh thyme, chopped (or 1 teaspoon dried thyme)
- 2 cloves garlic, minced
- 2 tablespoons olive oil
- 1 lemon, zested and juiced

  Salt and pepper to taste

DIRECTIONS

1. **Preheat Oven:** Preheat your oven to 400°F (200°C).
2. **Prepare Baking Dish:** Lightly grease a baking dish with olive oil or line it with parchment paper.
3. **Make Herb Crust:** In a bowl, combine almond flour, parsley, dill, thyme, minced garlic, lemon zest, salt, and pepper. Drizzle in olive oil and mix until the mixture resembles wet sand.
4. **Prepare Cod:** Place the cod fillets in the prepared baking dish. Squeeze lemon juice over the fillets and season with salt and pepper.
5. **Coat Cod:** Press the herb mixture onto the top of each cod fillet, ensuring an even coating.
6. **Bake:** Bake in the preheated oven for 12-15 minutes, or until the cod is cooked through and flakes easily with a fork.
7. **Serve:** Serve hot, garnished with lemon wedges if desired.

Nutrition Information (Per Serving)

Calories	280
Protein	30g
Fat	15g
Carbohydrates	10g
Fiber	3g
Sugar	1g

"Your health is a priority."

QUICK NOTES

TIPS FOR CUSTOMIZATION

- **Fish Options:** Substitute cod with other white fish like haddock, tilapia, or halibut.
- **Herbs:** Experiment with different herbs such as basil, oregano, or cilantro for varied flavors.
- **Add Vegetables:** Serve with a side of roasted vegetables or a fresh salad for a complete meal.

Why is this recipe good for PCOS?

- **High in Protein:** Cod is a lean source of protein, which helps stabilize blood sugar levels.
- **Low Carb:** This dish is low in carbohydrates, making it suitable for those managing insulin resistance.
- **Nutrient-Dense:** The use of fresh herbs adds antioxidants and anti-inflammatory properties, supporting overall health.
- **Healthy Fats:** Olive oil provides healthy fats that can help with hormone balance.

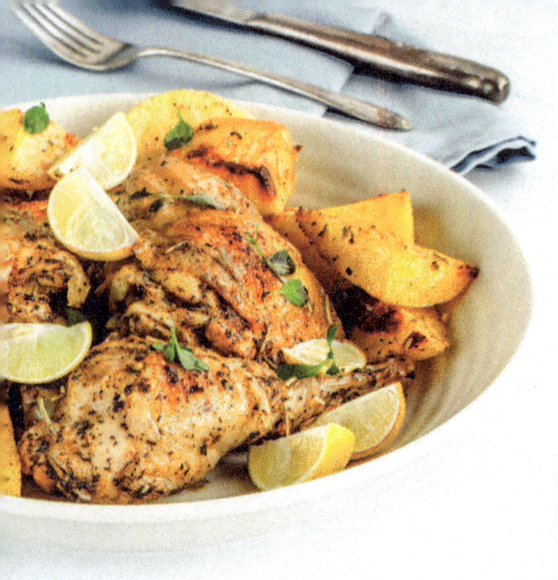

Lemon Herb Grilled Chicken

SERVING SIZE
Serves 4

INGREDIENTS

- 4 boneless, skinless chicken breasts (about 6 oz each)
- 1/4 cup olive oil
- 1/4 cup fresh lemon juice (about 2 lemons)
- 4 cloves garlic, minced
- 1 tablespoon fresh rosemary, chopped (or
- 1 teaspoon dried rosemary)
- 1 tablespoon fresh thyme, chopped (or 1 teaspoon dried thyme)
- 1 teaspoon salt
- 1/2 teaspoon black pepper
- Lemon wedges for serving (optional)

DIRECTIONS

1. **Prepare Marinade:** In a bowl, whisk together olive oil, lemon juice, minced garlic, rosemary, thyme, salt, and pepper.
2. **Marinate Chicken:** Place the chicken breasts in a resealable plastic bag or shallow dish. Pour the marinade over the chicken, ensuring it is well coated. Seal the bag or cover the dish and refrigerate for at least 30 minutes (up to 4 hours for more flavor).
3. **Preheat Grill:** Preheat your grill to medium-high heat.
4. **Grill Chicken:** Remove the chicken from the marinade and discard the marinade. Place the chicken on the grill and cook for about 6-7 minutes per side, or until the internal temperature reaches 165°F (75°C) and the chicken is cooked through.
5. **Serve:** Remove from the grill and let rest for a few minutes. Serve hot with lemon wedges on the side.

Nutrition Information (Per Serving)

Calories	280
Protein	30g
Fat	16g
Carbohydrates:	2g
Fiber	0g
Sugar	0g

"Be kind to yourself."

QUICK NOTES

TIPS FOR CUSTOMIZATION

- **Herbs:** Feel free to use other herbs like parsley, cilantro, or oregano for different flavor profiles.
- **Spice Level:** Add red pepper flakes or a dash of hot sauce to the marinade for a spicy kick.
- **Serving Suggestions:** Serve with a side of grilled vegetables or a fresh salad for a complete meal.

Why is this recipe good for PCOS?

- **High Protein:** Chicken is a lean source of protein, which helps stabilize blood sugar levels.
- **Low Carb:** This dish is low in carbohydrates, making it suitable for those managing insulin resistance.
- **Healthy Fats:** Olive oil provides healthy fats that can support hormone balance.
- **Nutrient-Dense:** The use of fresh herbs and lemon adds antioxidants and vitamins, promoting overall health.

Notes

Chapter 6.

PCOS - Friendly Snacks Ideas

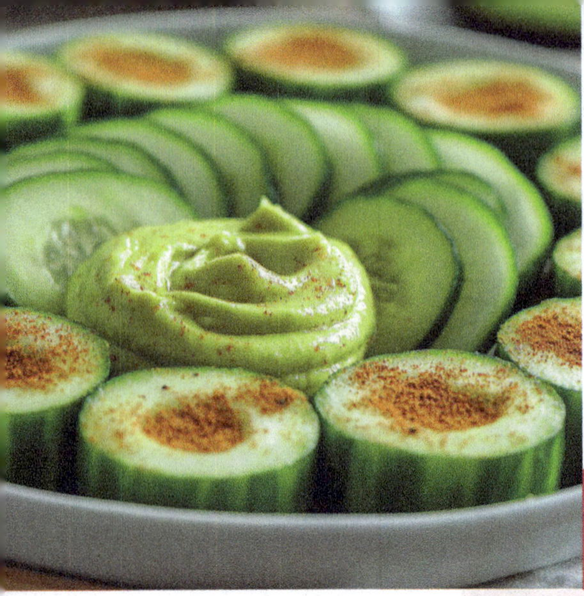

Avocado and Cucumber Bites

SERVING SIZE
Serves 4 (approx. 2-3 bites per person)

INGREDIENTS

- 1 large cucumber
- 1 ripe avocado
- 1 tablespoon lemon juice
- Salt and pepper to taste
- *Optional toppings* red pepper flakes, sesame seeds, or fresh herbs (e.g., cilantro or parsley)

DIRECTIONS

1. **Prepare Cucumber:** Slice the cucumber into 1/2-inch thick rounds and arrange them on a serving platter.
2. **Make Avocado Spread:** In a bowl, mash the ripe avocado with lemon juice, salt, and pepper until smooth. Adjust seasoning to taste.
3. **Assemble Bites:** Spoon a small amount of the avocado mixture onto each cucumber slice.
4. **Garnish:** If desired, sprinkle with red pepper flakes, sesame seeds, or fresh herbs for added flavor and presentation.
5. **Serve:** Enjoy immediately as a refreshing snack or appetizer.

Nutrition Information (Per Serving)

Calories	120
Protein	2g
Fat	10g
Carbohydrates	8g
Fiber	4g
Sugar	1g

QUICK NOTES

TIPS FOR CUSTOMIZATION

- **Add-ins:** Mix in diced tomatoes or red onion into the avocado spread for extra flavor.
- **Spice Level:** Add a pinch of cayenne pepper or hot sauce to the avocado for a spicy kick.
- **Herbs:** Experiment with different herbs like dill or chives for varied flavors.

Why is this recipe good for PCOS?

- **Healthy Fats:** Avocado provides healthy monounsaturated fats that can help with hormone balance.
- **Low Carb:** This snack is low in carbohydrates, making it suitable for those managing insulin resistance.
- **Nutrient-Dense:** Cucumbers are hydrating and low in calories, while avocados are rich in vitamins and minerals.
- **High Fiber:** The combination of avocado and cucumber provides fiber, which supports digestive health.

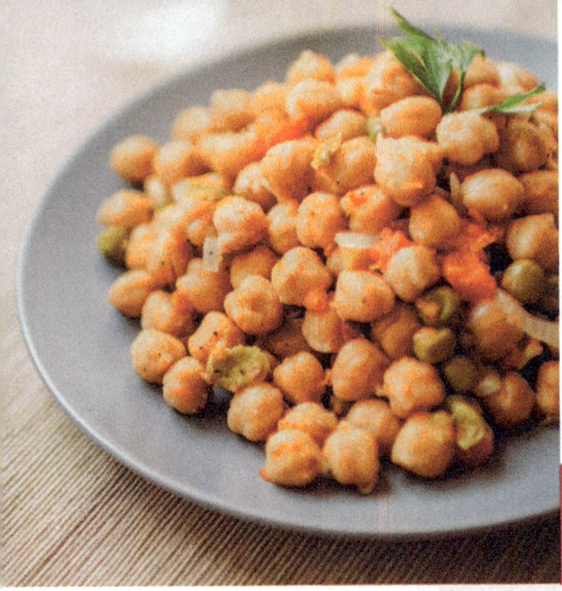

Roasted Chickpeas

SERVING SIZE
Serves 4

INGREDIENTS

- 1 can (15 oz) chickpeas, drained and rinsed
- 1 tablespoon olive oil
- 1 teaspoon salt
- 1 teaspoon smoked paprika (or your choice of spices, e.g., cumin, garlic powder, or chili powder)
- *Optional*
  1/2 teaspoon cayenne pepper (for heat)

DIRECTIONS

1. **Preheat Oven:** Preheat your oven to 400°F (200°C).
2. **Prepare Chickpeas:** After draining and rinsing the chickpeas, spread them out on a clean kitchen towel or paper towel. Pat them dry to remove excess moisture.
3. **Season Chickpeas:** In a bowl, toss the dried chickpeas with olive oil, salt, and your choice of spices until evenly coated.
4. **Roast:** Spread the seasoned chickpeas in a single layer on a baking sheet. Roast in the preheated oven for 20-30 minutes, shaking the pan halfway through, until they are golden brown and crispy.
5. **Cool and Serve:** Remove from the oven and let them cool slightly. They will continue to crisp up as they cool. Enjoy as a snack or topping for salads.

Nutrition Information (Per Serving)

Calories	150
Protein	6g
Fat	5g
Carbohydrates	22g
Fiber	6g
Sugar	1g

QUICK NOTES

TIPS FOR CUSTOMIZATION

- **Spices:** Experiment with different spice blends like curry powder, Italian seasoning, or ranch seasoning for varied flavors.
- **Sweet Version:** For a sweet snack, toss chickpeas with a little cinnamon and a low-carb sweetener before roasting.
- **Storage:** Store any leftovers in an airtight container at room temperature for up to 3 days, but they are best enjoyed fresh.

Why is this recipe good for PCOS?

- **High Fiber:** Chickpeas are rich in fiber, which helps regulate blood sugar levels and supports digestive health.
- **Plant-Based Protein:** They provide a good source of plant-based protein, beneficial for hormone balance.
- **Low Glycemic Index:** Roasted chickpeas have a low glycemic index, making them suitable for those managing insulin resistance.
- **Nutrient-Dense:** Chickpeas are packed with vitamins and minerals, promoting overall health.

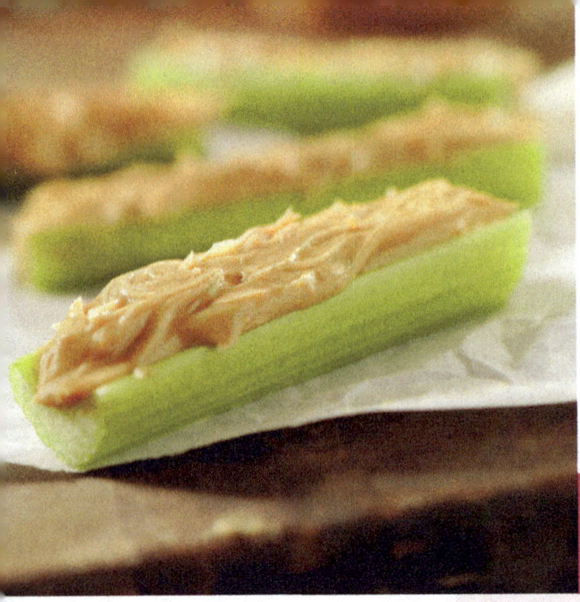

Nut Butter Celery Sticks

SERVING SIZE
Serves 2-3 (approx. 2-3 celery sticks per person

INGREDIENTS

- 4-6 celery stalks
- 1/2 cup almond butter, peanut butter, or any nut butter of your choice
- *Optional toppings* raisins, chia seeds, or shredded coconut

DIRECTIONS

1. **Prepare Celery:** Wash the celery stalks thoroughly and cut them into 3-4 inch pieces.
2. **Spread Nut Butter:** Using a knife or a spoon, spread a generous amount of nut butter into the groove of each celery stick.
3. **Add Toppings:** If desired, sprinkle toppings like raisins, chia seeds, or shredded coconut on top of the nut butter for added flavor and texture.
4. **Serve:** Enjoy immediately as a quick and nutritious snack.

Nutrition Information (Per Serving)

Calories	200
Protein	6g
Fat	16g
Carbohydrates	10g
Fiber	4g
Sugar	2g

QUICK NOTES

TIPS FOR CUSTOMIZATION

- **Nut Butter Variety:** Try different nut butters like cashew butter or sunflower seed butter for varied flavors.
- **Sweetness:** Drizzle a little honey or maple syrup over the nut butter for added sweetness (if not strictly low-carb).
- **Add Crunch:** Top with chopped nuts or seeds for extra crunch and nutrition.

Why is this recipe good for PCOS?

- **Healthy Fats:** Nut butter provides healthy fats that can help with hormone balance and satiety.
- **Low Carb:** This snack is low in carbohydrates, making it suitable for those managing insulin resistance.
- **High Fiber:** Celery is low in calories and high in fiber, which supports digestive health.
- **Nutrient-Dense:** The combination of nut butter and celery offers vitamins, minerals, and antioxidants, promoting overall health.

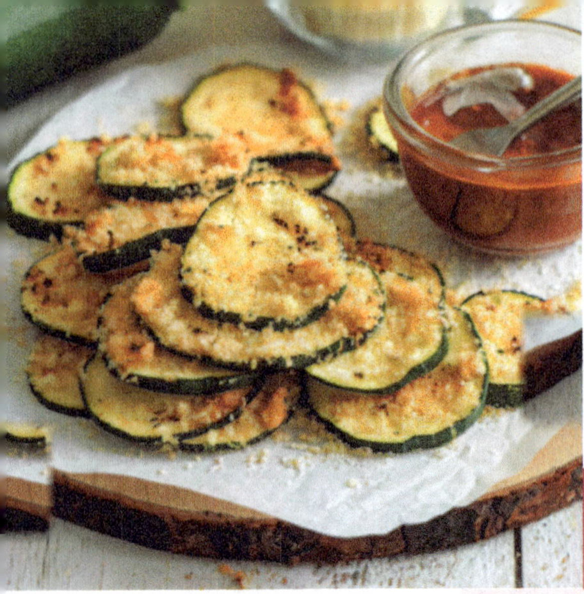

Zucchini Chips

SERVING SIZE
Serves 4

INGREDIENTS

- 2 medium zucchinis
- 2 tablespoons olive oil
  1 teaspoon salt
- 1/2 teaspoon garlic powder (optional)
- 1/2 teaspoon smoked paprika (optional)
- Freshly ground black pepper to taste

DIRECTIONS

1. **Preheat Oven:** Preheat your oven to 225°F (110°C).
2. **Prepare Zucchini:** Wash the zucchinis and slice them thinly (about 1/8 inch thick) using a mandoline or a sharp knife.
3. **Season Zucchini:** In a large bowl, toss the zucchini slices with olive oil, salt, garlic powder, smoked paprika, and black pepper until evenly coated.
4. **Arrange on Baking Sheet:** Place the zucchini slices in a single layer on a baking sheet lined with parchment paper. Make sure they are not overlapping to ensure even cooking.
5. **Bake:** Bake in the preheated oven for 2-3 hours, flipping the chips halfway through, until they are crispy and golden brown. Keep an eye on them to prevent burning.
6. **Cool and Serve:** Remove from the oven and let the chips cool completely. They will continue to crisp up as they cool. Enjoy as a snack!

Nutrition Information (Per Serving)

Calories	100
Protein	2g
Fat	7g
Carbohydrates	8g
Fiber	2g
Sugar	2g

QUICK NOTES

TIPS FOR CUSTOMIZATION

- **Spices:** Experiment with different spices like Italian seasoning, chili powder, or nutritional yeast for added flavor.
- **Dipping Sauce:** Serve with a dairy-free dip like hummus or guacamole for extra flavor.
- **Storage:** Store any leftovers in an airtight container at room temperature for up to 3 days, but they are best enjoyed fresh.

Why is this recipe good for PCOS?

- **Low Carb:** Zucchini chips are low in carbohydrates, making them suitable for those managing insulin resistance.
- **High Fiber:** Zucchini is high in fiber, which supports digestive health and helps regulate blood sugar levels.
- **Nutrient-Dense:** Zucchini is rich in vitamins and minerals, promoting overall health.
- **Healthy Fats:** The use of olive oil provides healthy fats that can support hormone balance.

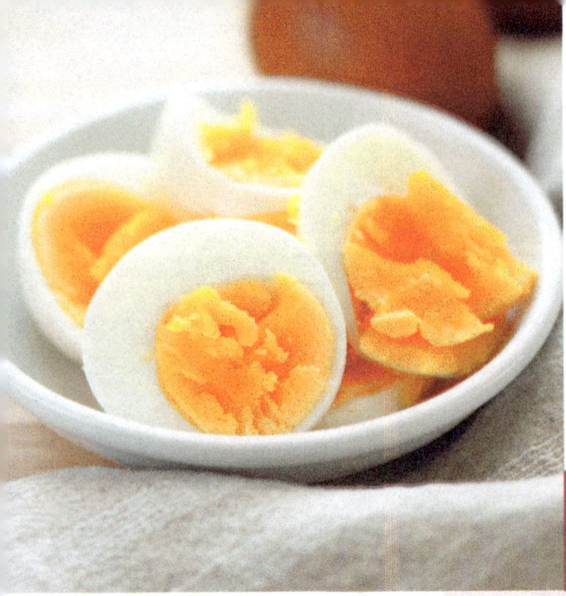

Hard-Boiled Eggs

SERVING SIZE
Serves 3 (2 eggs per serving)

INGREDIENTS

- 6 large eggs

DIRECTIONS

1. **Place Eggs in Pot:** Place the eggs in a single layer in a saucepan or pot. Add enough water to cover the eggs by about an inch.
2. **Boil Water:** Bring the water to a boil over medium-high heat.
3. **Simmer:** Once the water reaches a rolling boil, cover the pot with a lid and remove it from heat. Let the eggs sit in the hot water for 7-12 minutes, depending on how well-done you prefer the yolks (7 minutes for slightly soft yolks, 12 minutes for fully hard-boiled).
4. **Cool Eggs:** After the time is up, carefully transfer the eggs to a bowl of ice water or run them under cold water for several minutes to stop the cooking process.
5. **Peel and Serve:** Once cooled, gently tap the eggs on a hard surface to crack the shell, then peel under running water for easier removal. Enjoy as a snack or use in salads and other dishes.

Nutrition Information (Per Serving)

Calories	140
Protein	12g
Fat	10g
Carbohydrates	1g
Fiber	0g
Sugar	0g

QUICK NOTES

TIPS FOR CUSTOMIZATION

- **Seasoning:** Sprinkle with salt, pepper, or your favorite seasoning blend for added flavor.
- **Deviled Eggs:** Mash the yolks with avocado or mustard for a healthier deviled egg option.
- **Storage:** Store hard-boiled eggs in the refrigerator for up to one week.

Why is this recipe good for PCOS?

- **High Protein:** Eggs are an excellent source of high-quality protein, which helps stabilize blood sugar levels.
- **Low Carb:** Hard-boiled eggs are low in carbohydrates, making them suitable for those managing insulin resistance.
- **Nutrient-Dense:** Eggs are rich in vitamins and minerals, including vitamin D, B vitamins, and selenium, promoting overall health.
- **Healthy Fats:** The fats in eggs can help with satiety and hormone balance.

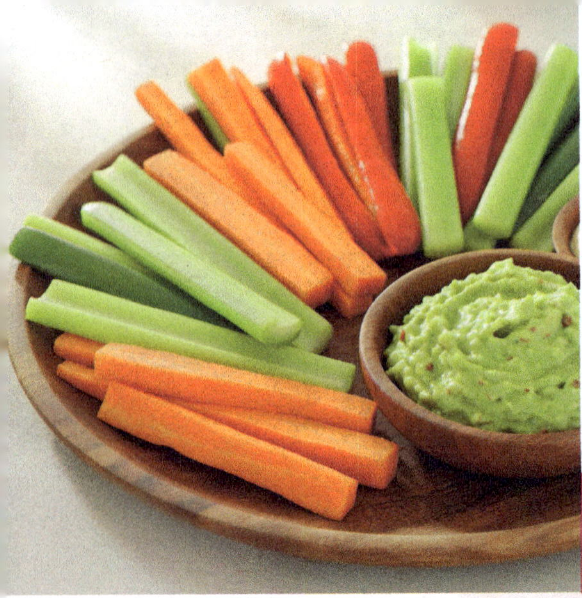

Guacamole with Veggie Sticks

SERVING SIZE
Serves 4

INGREDIENTS

For the Guacamole

- 2 ripe avocados
- 1 small lime, juiced
- 1 small garlic clove, minced
- 1/4 small red onion, finely chopped
- 1 small tomato, diced (optional)
  Salt and pepper to taste
  Fresh cilantro, chopped (optional)

For the Veggie Sticks

- 1 cucumber, cut into sticks
- 2-3 carrots, cut into sticks
- 1 bell pepper, cut into strips
- 1 celery stalk, cut into sticks

DIRECTIONS

1. **Prepare Guacamole:** In a bowl, mash the avocados with a fork until smooth or chunky, depending on your preference. Add lime juice, minced garlic, chopped red onion, diced tomato (if using), salt, and pepper. Mix well to combine. Stir in chopped cilantro if desired. Prepare
2. **Veggie Sticks:** Wash and cut the vegetables into sticks or strips. Arrange them on a serving platter.
3. **Serve:** Serve the guacamole in a bowl alongside the veggie sticks for dipping.

Nutrition Information (Per Serving)

Calories	180
Protein	3g
Fat	15g
Carbohydrates	10g
Fiber	7g
Sugar	2g

QUICK NOTES

TIPS FOR CUSTOMIZATION

- **Spice Level:** Add diced jalapeños or a pinch of cayenne pepper for a spicy kick.
- **Add-ins:** Mix in other ingredients like corn, black beans, or diced mango for added flavor and texture.
- **Storage:** Store any leftover guacamole in an airtight container with plastic wrap pressed against the surface to minimize browning.

Why is this recipe good for PCOS?

- **Healthy Fats:** Avocado provides healthy monounsaturated fats that can help with hormone balance.
- **Low Carb:** This snack is low in carbohydrates, making it suitable for those managing insulin resistance.
- **High Fiber:** The combination of avocado and vegetables offers fiber, which supports digestive health.
- **Nutrient-Dense:** The ingredients are rich in vitamins, minerals, and antioxidants, promoting overall health.

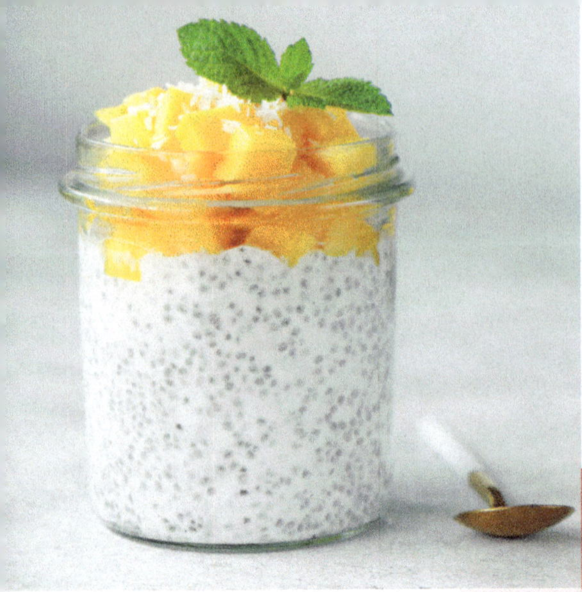

Chia Seed Pudding

SERVING SIZE
Serves 2

INGREDIENTS

- 1/4 cup chia seeds
- 1 cup almond milk (or any dairy-free milk of your choice)
- 1 tablespoon maple syrup or honey (optional, adjust to taste)
- 1/2 teaspoon vanilla extract
- Fresh fruit for topping (e.g., berries, banana, or mango)
- Nuts or seeds for topping (optional)

DIRECTIONS

1. **Combine Ingredients:** In a bowl or jar, mix together chia seeds, almond milk, maple syrup (if using), and vanilla extract. Stir well to combine.
2. **Let it Sit:** Allow the mixture to sit for about 5 minutes, then stir again to prevent clumping.
3. **Refrigerate:** Cover the bowl or jar and refrigerate for at least 2 hours, or overnight, until the chia seeds have absorbed the liquid and the pudding has thickened.
4. **Serve:** Once thickened, give the pudding a good stir. Serve in bowls or jars topped with fresh fruit and nuts or seeds if desired.

Nutrition Information (Per Serving)

Calories	180
Protein	5g
Fat	9g
Carbohydrates	22g
Fiber	10g
Sugar	4g

QUICK NOTES

TIPS FOR CUSTOMIZATION

- **Flavor Variations:** Add cocoa powder for chocolate chia pudding or matcha powder for a green tea flavor.
- **Fruit:** Mix in pureed fruit like banana or mango for added sweetness and flavor.
- **Toppings:** Experiment with different toppings like coconut flakes, granola, or nut butter for added texture and flavor.

Why is this recipe good for PCOS?

- **High Fiber:** Chia seeds are rich in fiber, which helps regulate blood sugar levels and supports digestive health.
- **Healthy Fats:** They provide omega-3 fatty acids, which can help reduce inflammation and support hormone balance.
- **Low Glycemic Index:** Chia seed pudding has a low glycemic index, making it suitable for those managing insulin resistance.
- **Nutrient-Dense:** This pudding is packed with vitamins, minerals, and antioxidants, promoting overall health.

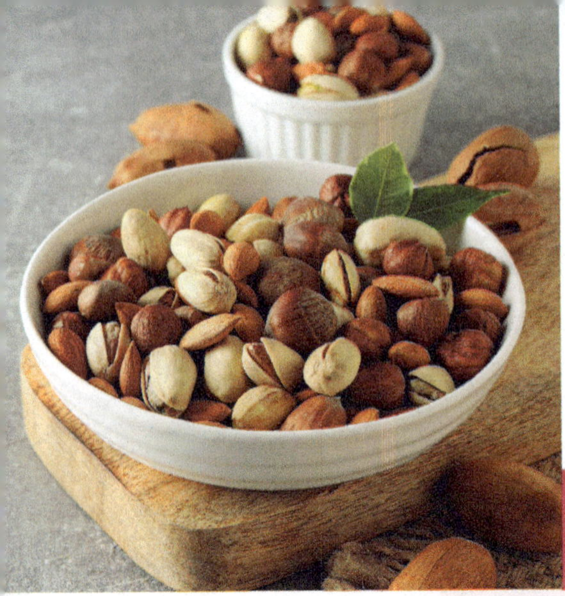

Olives and Nuts Mix

SERVING SIZE
Serves 4

INGREDIENTS

- 1 cup mixed olives (green, black, or kalamata), pitted
- 1 cup mixed nuts (e.g., almonds, walnuts, pecans, or cashews)
- 1 tablespoon olive oil (optional)
- 1 teaspoon dried herbs (e.g., oregano, thyme, or rosemary)
- 1/2 teaspoon garlic powder (optional)
- Salt and pepper to taste
- *Optional*
  Red pepper flakes for heat

DIRECTIONS

1. **Prepare Olives:** If using whole olives, ensure they are pitted. You can slice them in half for easier snacking.
2. **Mix Ingredients:** In a large bowl, combine the mixed olives and nuts. If desired, drizzle with olive oil and sprinkle with dried herbs, garlic powder, salt, and pepper. Toss to combine.
3. **Adjust Seasoning:** Taste the mixture and adjust the seasoning as needed. Add red pepper flakes if you prefer a spicy kick.
4. **Serve:** Serve immediately as a snack or appetizer, or store in an airtight container for later.

Nutrition Information (Per Serving)

Calories	200
Protein	5g
Fat	18g
Carbohydrates	8g
Fiber	3g
Sugar	1g

QUICK NOTES

TIPS FOR CUSTOMIZATION

- **Nut Variety:** Use your favorite nuts or seeds, and consider adding roasted or spiced varieties for extra flavor.
- **Olive Variety:** Experiment with different types of olives for varied taste and texture.
- **Add-ins:** Include dried fruits like cranberries or apricots for a sweet contrast (note that this will increase the sugar content).

Why is this recipe good for PCOS?

- **Healthy Fats:** Both olives and nuts are rich in healthy fats, which can help with hormone balance and satiety.
- **Low Carb:** This snack is low in carbohydrates, making it suitable for those managing insulin resistance.
- **Nutrient-Dense:** Olives and nuts provide a variety of vitamins, minerals, and antioxidants, promoting overall health.
- **High Fiber:** The combination of nuts and olives offers fiber, which supports digestive health.

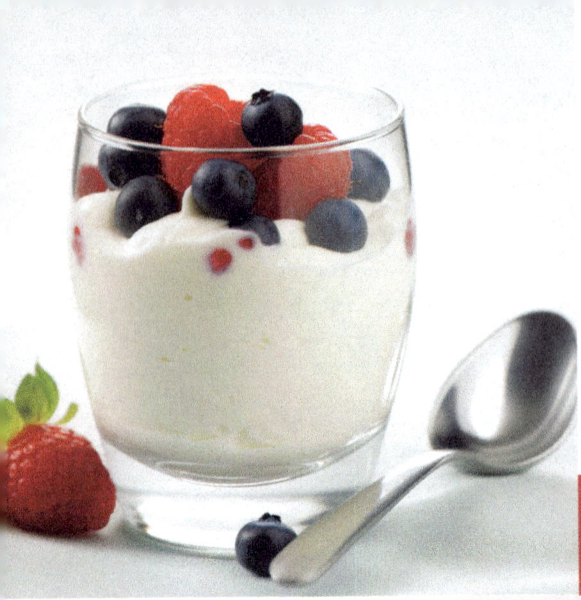

Coconut Yogurt with Berries

SERVING SIZE
Serves 2

INGREDIENTS

- 1 cup dairy-free coconut yogurt (store-bought or homemade)
- 1/2 cup fresh berries (e.g., strawberries, blueberries, raspberries, or blackberries)
- 1 tablespoon chia seeds (optional, for added fiber)
- 1 tablespoon maple syrup or honey (optional, adjust to taste)
- 1/4 teaspoon vanilla extract (optional)
- Nuts or seeds for topping (optional)

DIRECTIONS

1. **Prepare Yogurt Base:** In a bowl, add the coconut yogurt. If using, stir in the maple syrup or honey and vanilla extract until well combined.
2. **Add Chia Seeds:** If desired, mix in chia seeds for added texture and nutrition.
3. **Top with Berries:** Gently fold in the fresh berries or layer them on top of the yogurt.
4. **Serve:** Serve immediately, topped with additional nuts or seeds if desired.

Nutrition Information (Per Serving)

Calories	180
Protein	3g
Fat	10g
Carbohydrates	20g
Fiber	5g
Sugar	6g

QUICK NOTES

TIPS FOR CUSTOMIZATION

- **Berry Variety:** Use any combination of fresh or frozen berries based on your preference and availability.
- **Add-ins:** Mix in other toppings like shredded coconut, granola, or nut butter for extra flavor and texture.
- **Sweetness:** Adjust the sweetness by adding more or less maple syrup or honey according to your taste.

Why is this recipe good for PCOS?

- **Dairy-Free:** Coconut yogurt is a great alternative for those avoiding dairy, which can be beneficial for some individuals with PCOS.
- **Healthy Fats:** Coconut yogurt provides healthy fats that can help with hormone balance and satiety.
- **Low Glycemic Index:** This dessert is low in sugar and has a low glycemic index, making it suitable for those managing insulin resistance.
- **Nutrient-Dense:** Berries are rich in antioxidants, vitamins, and minerals, promoting overall health.

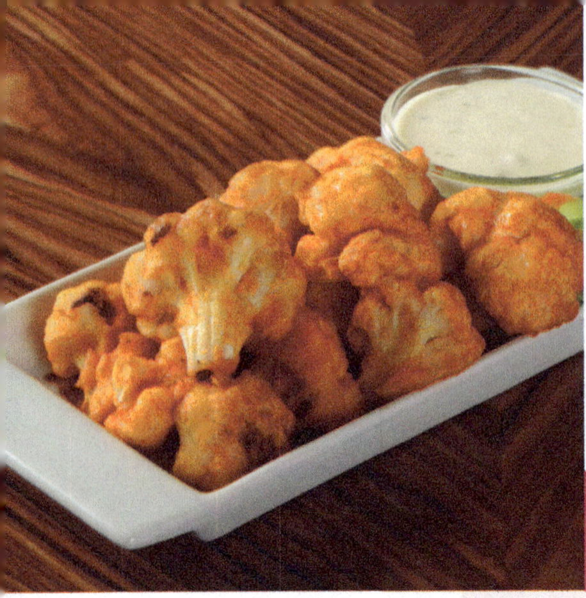

Spicy Roasted Cauliflower Bites

SERVING SIZE
Serves 4

INGREDIENTS

- 1 medium head of cauliflower, cut into bite-sized florets
- 2 tablespoons olive oil
- 1 teaspoon smoked paprika
- 1 teaspoon garlic powder
- 1/2 teaspoon cayenne pepper (adjust to taste)
- 1 teaspoon salt
- 1/2 teaspoon black pepper
- *Optional*
  1 tablespoon nutritional yeast (for a cheesy flavor)

DIRECTIONS

1. **Preheat Oven:** Preheat your oven to 425°F (220°C).
2. **Prepare Cauliflower:** In a large bowl, combine the cauliflower florets with olive oil, smoked paprika, garlic powder, cayenne pepper, salt, and black pepper. Toss until the cauliflower is evenly coated.
3. **Arrange on Baking Sheet:** Spread the seasoned cauliflower in a single layer on a baking sheet lined with parchment paper.
4. **Roast:** Roast in the preheated oven for 25-30 minutes, or until the cauliflower is tender and golden brown, stirring halfway through for even cooking.
5. **Add Nutritional Yeast:** If using, sprinkle nutritional yeast over the cauliflower bites during the last 5 minutes of roasting for added flavor.
6. **Serve:** Remove from the oven and let cool slightly before serving. Enjoy as a snack or side dish!

Nutrition Information (Per Serving)

Calories	120
Protein	3g
Fat	8g
Carbohydrates	10g
Fiber	4g
Sugar	2g

QUICK NOTES

TIPS FOR CUSTOMIZATION

- **Spice Level:** Adjust the amount of cayenne pepper based on your spice preference. You can also add chili powder or hot sauce for extra heat.
- **Add-ins:** Mix in other vegetables like broccoli or carrots for a colorful medley.
- **Dipping Sauce:** Serve with a dairy-free dip like tahini sauce or hummus for added flavor.

Why is this recipe good for PCOS?

- **Low Carb:** Cauliflower is low in carbohydrates, making it suitable for those managing insulin resistance.
- **High Fiber:** Cauliflower is high in fiber, which supports digestive health and helps regulate blood sugar levels.
- **Nutrient-Dense:** This dish is rich in vitamins and minerals, promoting overall health.
- **Healthy Fats:** The use of olive oil provides healthy fats that can support hormone balance.

Notes

1.

Chapter

PCOS - Friendly

Dessert Ideas

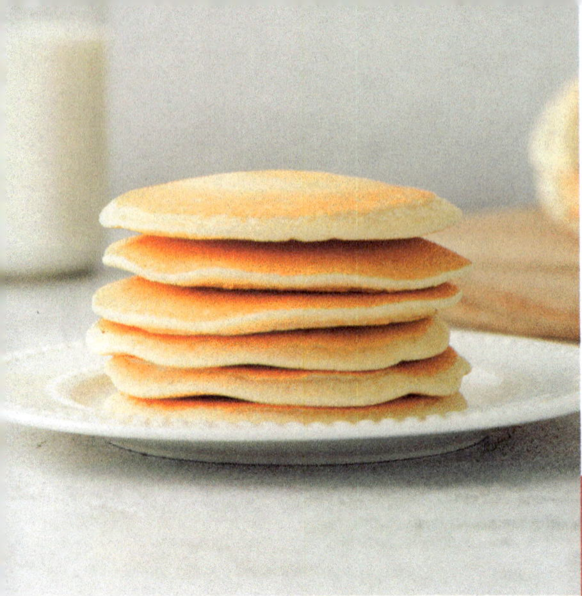

Coconut Flour Pancakes

SERVING SIZE
Serves 2 (makes about 4-6 pancakes)

INGREDIENTS

- 1/4 cup coconut flour
- 4 large eggs
- 1/4 cup almond milk (or any dairy-free milk)
- 1 tablespoon coconut oil (melted) or another oil
- 1 tablespoon low-carb sweetener (e.g., erythritol or stevia)
- 1/2 teaspoon baking powder
- 1/4 teaspoon salt
- *Optional*
  1/2 teaspoon vanilla extract

DIRECTIONS

1. **Mix Dry Ingredients:** In a bowl, combine coconut flour, baking powder, and salt. Mix well to ensure there are no lumps.
2. **Combine Wet Ingredients:** In another bowl, whisk together the eggs, almond milk, melted coconut oil, low-carb sweetener, and vanilla extract (if using).
3. **Combine Mixtures:** Gradually add the dry ingredients to the wet ingredients, stirring until well combined. Let the batter sit for a few minutes to thicken.
4. **Preheat Pan:** Heat a non-stick skillet or griddle over medium heat. Lightly grease with coconut oil or cooking spray.
5. **Cook Pancakes:** Pour about 1/4 cup of batter onto the skillet for each pancake. Cook for 2-3 minutes until bubbles form on the surface, then flip and cook for another 2-3 minutes until golden brown.
6. **Serve:** Serve warm with your favorite toppings, such as fresh berries, sugar-free syrup, or nut butter.

Nutrition Information (Per Serving)

Calories	250
Protein	10g
Fat	18g
Carbohydrates	10g
Fiber	5g
Sugar	1g

QUICK NOTES

TIPS FOR CUSTOMIZATION

- **Add-ins:** Mix in blueberries, chocolate chips, or nuts for added flavor and texture.
- **Toppings:** Top with sliced bananas, almond butter, or a sprinkle of cinnamon for extra taste.
- **Storage:** Store any leftovers in an airtight container in the refrigerator for up to 3 days. Reheat in a skillet or microwave.

Why is this recipe good for PCOS?

- **Low Carb:** Coconut flour is low in carbohydrates, making it suitable for those managing insulin resistance.
- **High Fiber:** Coconut flour is high in fiber, which supports digestive health and helps regulate blood sugar levels.
- **Healthy Fats:** The use of coconut oil provides healthy fats that can support hormone balance.
- **Nutrient-Dense:** This recipe is rich in vitamins and minerals, promoting overall health.

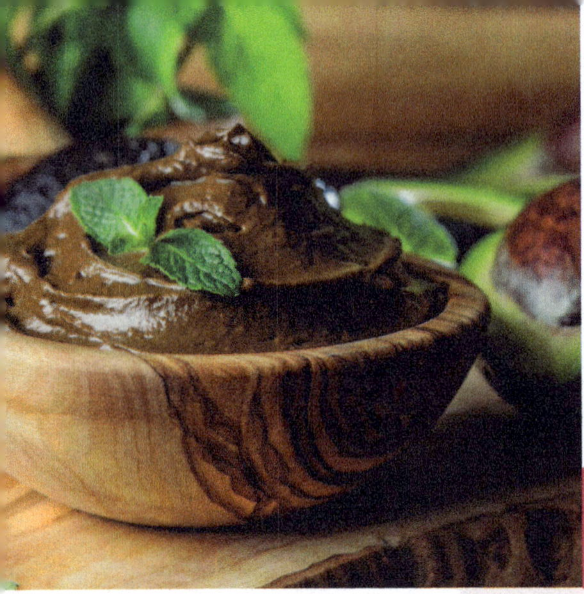

Avocado Chocolate Mousse

SERVING SIZE
Serves 4

INGREDIENTS

- 2 ripe avocados
- 1/4 cup unsweetened cocoa powder
- 1/4 cup almond milk (or any dairy-free milk)
- 1/4 cup low-carb sweetener (e.g., erythritol, stevia, or maple syrup)
- 1 teaspoon vanilla extract
- A pinch of salt

DIRECTIONS

1. **Prepare Avocados:** Cut the avocados in half, remove the pit, and scoop the flesh into a food processor or blender.
2. **Add Ingredients:** Add cocoa powder, almond milk, low-carb sweetener, vanilla extract, and a pinch of salt to the food processor.
3. **Blend:** Blend until smooth and creamy, scraping down the sides as needed. Taste and adjust sweetness if necessary.
4. **Chill:** Transfer the mousse to serving bowls or cups and refrigerate for at least 30 minutes to allow it to set and chill.
5. **Serve:** Serve chilled, optionally topped with fresh berries, nuts, or a dollop of coconut whipped cream.

Nutrition Information (Per Serving)

Calories	180
Protein	3g
Fat	12g
Carbohydrates	15g
Fiber	7g
Sugar	2g

QUICK NOTES

TIPS FOR CUSTOMIZATION

- **Flavor Variations:** Add a teaspoon of instant coffee or espresso powder for a mocha flavor.
- **Toppings:** Top with sliced bananas, shredded coconut, or chopped nuts for added texture.
- **Storage:** Store any leftovers in an airtight container in the refrigerator for up to 2 days.

Why is this recipe good for PCOS?

- **Healthy Fats:** Avocados provide healthy monounsaturated fats that can help with hormone balance and satiety.
- **Low Carb:** This dessert is low in carbohydrates, making it suitable for those managing insulin resistance.
- **Nutrient-Dense:** Avocados are rich in vitamins, minerals, and antioxidants, promoting overall health.
- **High Fiber:** The fiber content helps regulate blood sugar levels and supports digestive health.

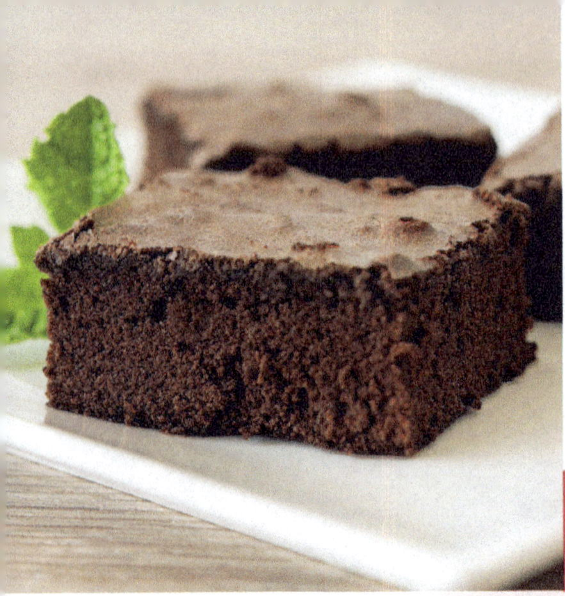

Coconut Flour Brownies

SERVING SIZE
Serves 9

INGREDIENTS

- 1/2 cup coconut flour
- 1/2 cup unsweetened cocoa powder
- 1/2 cup low-carb sweetener (e.g., erythritol or stevia)
- 1/2 teaspoon baking powder
- 1/4 teaspoon salt
- 4 large eggs
- 1/2 cup coconut oil (melted) or unsalted butter (dairy-free if needed)
- 1 teaspoon vanilla extract
- *Optional*
  1/2 cup sugar-free chocolate chips or nuts for added texture

DIRECTIONS

1. **Preheat Oven:** Preheat your oven to 350°F (175°C). Grease an 8x8-inch baking pan or line it with parchment paper.
2. **Mix Dry Ingredients:** In a large bowl, combine coconut flour, cocoa powder, low-carb sweetener, baking powder, and salt. Mix well to ensure there are no lumps.
3. **Combine Wet Ingredients:** In another bowl, whisk together the eggs, melted coconut oil, and vanilla extract until well combined.
4. **Combine Mixtures:** Gradually add the wet ingredients to the dry ingredients, stirring until fully combined. If using, fold in chocolate chips or nuts.
5. **Pour Batter:** Pour the brownie batter into the prepared baking pan and spread it evenly.
6. **Bake:** Bake in the preheated oven for 20-25 minutes, or until a toothpick inserted in the center comes out clean or with a few moist crumbs.
   Cool and
7. **Serve:** Allow the brownies to cool in the pan for about 10 minutes before slicing into squares. Enjoy!

Nutrition Information (Per Serving)

Calories	150
Protein	4g
Fat	10g
Carbohydrates	12g
Fiber	5g
Sugar	1g

QUICK NOTES

TIPS FOR CUSTOMIZATION

- **Add-ins:** Mix in chopped nuts, sugar-free chocolate chips, or dried fruit for added flavor and texture.
- **Frosting:** Top with a dairy-free frosting or a drizzle of melted dark chocolate for extra indulgence.
- **Storage:** Store leftovers in an airtight container at room temperature for up to 3 days or in the refrigerator for up to a week.

Why is this recipe good for PCOS?

- **Low Carb:** Coconut flour is low in carbohydrates, making it suitable for those managing insulin resistance.
- **High Fiber:** Coconut flour is high in fiber, which supports digestive health and helps regulate blood sugar levels.
- **Healthy Fats:** The use of coconut oil provides healthy fats that can support hormone balance.
- **Nutrient-Dense:** This recipe is rich in vitamins and minerals, promoting overall health.

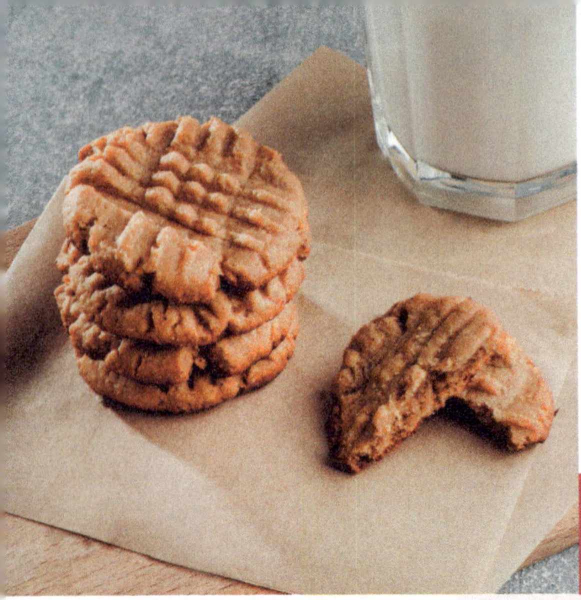

Almond Butter Cookies

SERVING SIZE
Serves 12 (approx. 2 cookies per serving)

INGREDIENTS

- 1 cup almond butter (smooth or crunchy)
- 1/2 cup low-carb sweetener (e.g., erythritol or stevia)
- 1 large egg
- 1 teaspoon vanilla extract
- 1/2 teaspoon baking soda
- 1/4 teaspoon salt
- *Optional*
  1/2 cup sugar-free chocolate chips or chopped nuts for added texture

DIRECTIONS

1. **Preheat Oven:** Preheat your oven to 350°F (175°C). Line a baking sheet with parchment paper.
2. **Mix Ingredients:** In a large bowl, combine almond butter, low-carb sweetener, egg, vanilla extract, baking soda, and salt. Mix until well combined and smooth.
3. **Add Optional Ingredients:** If using, fold in chocolate chips or chopped nuts.
4. **Form Cookies:** Scoop tablespoon-sized portions of dough and roll them into balls. Place them on the prepared baking sheet, spacing them about 2 inches apart. Flatten each ball slightly with the back of a fork or your hand.
5. **Bake:** Bake in the preheated oven for 10-12 minutes, or until the edges are lightly golden. The cookies will firm up as they cool.
6. **Cool and Serve:** Allow the cookies to cool on the baking sheet for a few minutes before transferring them to a wire rack to cool completely.

Nutrition Information (Per Serving)

Calories	150
Protein	4g
Fat	12g
Carbohydrates	6g
Fiber	2g
Sugar	1g

QUICK NOTES

TIPS FOR CUSTOMIZATION

- **Flavor Variations:** Add a pinch of cinnamon or cocoa powder for different flavor profiles.
- **Nut Butter:** Substitute almond butter with other nut butters like peanut butter or cashew butter if desired.
- **Storage:** Store cookies in an airtight container at room temperature for up to 5 days or in the refrigerator for up to 2 weeks.

Why is this recipe good for PCOS?

- **Low Carb:** These cookies are low in carbohydrates, making them suitable for those managing insulin resistance.
- **Healthy Fats:** Almond butter provides healthy fats that can help with hormone balance and satiety.
- **High Protein:** The combination of almond butter and egg offers a good source of protein, which helps stabilize blood sugar levels.
- **Nutrient-Dense:** Almonds are rich in vitamins, minerals, and antioxidants, promoting overall health.

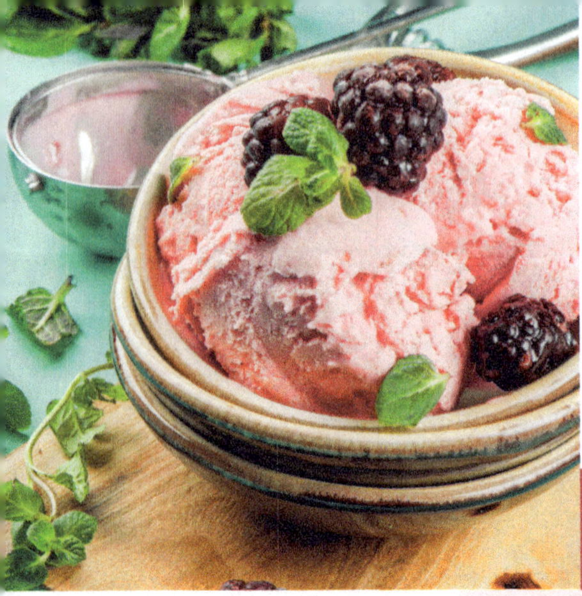

Sugar-Free Berry Sorbet

SERVING SIZE
Serves 4

INGREDIENTS

- 2 cups mixed berries (e.g., strawberries, blueberries, raspberries, or blackberries), fresh or frozen
- 1/4 cup water
- 1-2 tablespoons low-carb sweetener (e.g., erythritol, stevia, or monk fruit), adjust to taste
- 1 tablespoon lemon juice (optional)

DIRECTIONS

1. **Blend Ingredients:** In a blender or food processor, combine the mixed berries, water, low-carb sweetener, and lemon juice (if using). Blend until smooth.
2. **Taste and Adjust:** Taste the mixture and adjust the sweetness if needed by adding more sweetener.
3. **Freeze:** Pour the berry mixture into a shallow dish or ice cream maker. If using a shallow dish, spread it out evenly. Freeze for about 2-3 hours, or until firm.
4. **Stir Occasionally:** If using a shallow dish, stir the mixture every 30 minutes to break up any ice crystals until it reaches a sorbet-like consistency.
5. **Serve:** Once frozen, scoop the sorbet into bowls and serve immediately. If it's too hard, let it sit at room temperature for a few minutes to soften before serving.

Nutrition Information (Per Serving)

Calories	50
Protein	1g
Fat	0g
Carbohydrates	12g
Fiber	3g
Sugar	2g

QUICK NOTES

TIPS FOR CUSTOMIZATION

- **Berry Variety:** Use any combination of berries based on your preference and availability.
- **Add-ins:** Mix in a splash of vanilla extract or a pinch of salt for enhanced flavor.
- **Storage:** Store any leftovers in an airtight container in the freezer for up to 1 week. Let it sit at room temperature for a few minutes before scooping.

Why is this recipe good for PCOS?

- **Low Carb:** This sorbet is low in carbohydrates, making it suitable for those managing insulin resistance.
- **Nutrient-Dense:** Berries are rich in antioxidants, vitamins, and minerals, promoting overall health.
- **No Added Sugar:** Using a low-carb sweetener helps keep the sugar content low, which is beneficial for blood sugar management.
- **Hydrating:** The high water content in berries helps keep you hydrated, especially during warmer months.

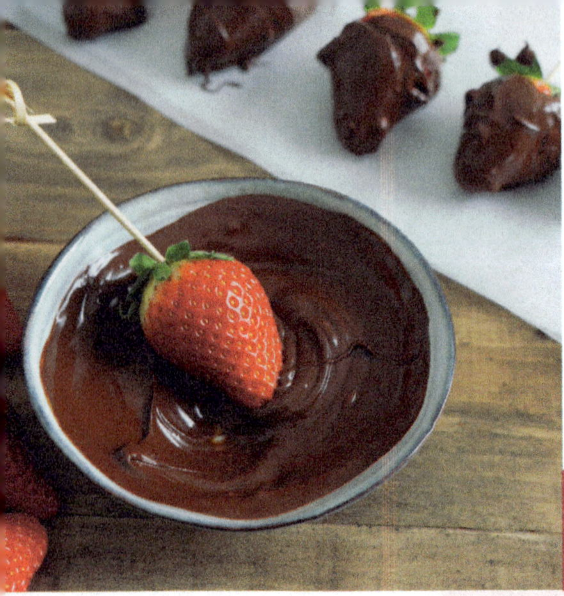

Dark Chocolate Dipped Strawberries

SERVING SIZE
Serves 4 (approx. 2 strawberries per serving

INGREDIENTS

- 1 cup fresh strawberries, washed and dried
- 1/2 cup dark chocolate chips (sugar-free or dairy-free, if needed)
- 1 teaspoon coconut oil (optional, for smoother chocolate)
- *Optional toppings* chopped nuts, shredded coconut, or sea salt

DIRECTIONS

1. **Prepare Strawberries:** Make sure the strawberries are completely dry after washing, as water can cause the chocolate to seize.
2. **Melt Chocolate:** In a microwave-safe bowl, combine dark chocolate chips and coconut oil (if using). Microwave in 30-second intervals, stirring in between, until the chocolate is fully melted and smooth.
3. **Dip Strawberries:** Hold each strawberry by the stem and dip it into the melted chocolate, allowing any excess chocolate to drip off. Place the dipped strawberry on a parchment-lined baking sheet.
4. **Add Toppings:** If desired, sprinkle chopped nuts, shredded coconut, or a pinch of sea salt on top of the chocolate before it sets.
5. **Chill:** Place the baking sheet in the refrigerator for about 30 minutes, or until the chocolate has hardened.
6. **Serve:** Enjoy the chocolate-dipped strawberries immediately or store them in an airtight container in the refrigerator for up to 2 days.

Nutrition Information (Per Serving)

Calories	120
Protein	2g
Fat	8g
Carbohydrates	10g
Fiber	3g
Sugar	2g

QUICK NOTES

TIPS FOR CUSTOMIZATION

- **Chocolate Variety:** Use different types of chocolate, such as milk chocolate or white chocolate (sugar-free), based on your preference.
- **Fruit Options:** Try dipping other fruits like bananas, apple slices, or orange segments for variety.
- **Storage:** Store any leftovers in an airtight container in the refrigerator for up to 2 days.

Why is this recipe good for PCOS?

- **Low Sugar:** Using sugar-free chocolate helps keep the sugar content low, which is beneficial for blood sugar management.
- **Antioxidants:** Dark chocolate is rich in antioxidants, which can help reduce inflammation and support overall health.
- **Nutrient-Dense:** Strawberries are low in calories and high in vitamins, minerals, and fiber, promoting overall health.
- **Healthy Fats:** The use of coconut oil adds healthy fats that can support hormone balance.

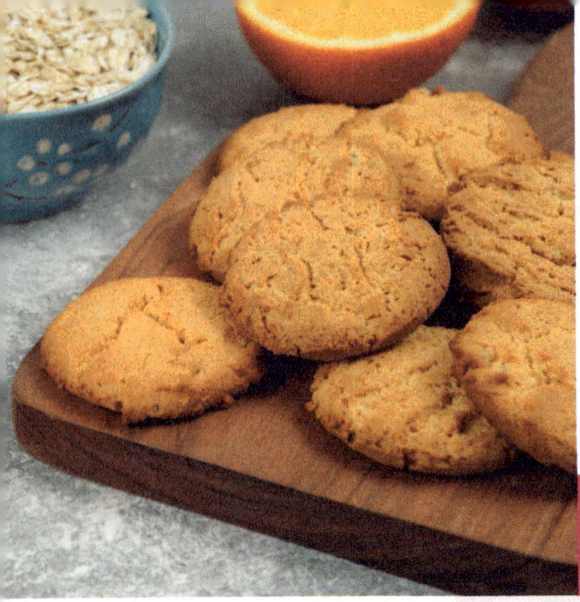

Banana Oatmeal Cookies

SERVING SIZE
Serves 4 (approx. 2 cookies per serving)

INGREDIENTS

- 2 ripe bananas, mashed
- 1 cup rolled oats (gluten-free if needed)
  1/4 cup almond butter or peanut butter
- 1/4 cup low-carb sweetener (e.g., erythritol or stevia, optional)
- 1/2 teaspoon vanilla extract
- 1/2 teaspoon cinnamon (optional)
- 1/4 teaspoon salt
- *Optional add-ins*
  1/4 cup sugar-free chocolate chips, nuts, or dried fruit

DIRECTIONS

1. **Preheat Oven:** Preheat your oven to 350°F (175°C). Line a baking sheet with parchment paper.
2. **Mix Ingredients:** In a large bowl, combine the mashed bananas, rolled oats, almond butter, low-carb sweetener (if using), vanilla extract, cinnamon, and salt. Mix until well combined. If using, fold in chocolate chips, nuts, or dried fruit.
3. **Form Cookies:** Scoop tablespoon-sized portions of the dough and place them on the prepared baking sheet, flattening them slightly with the back of a spoon
4. **Bake:** Bake in the preheated oven for 10-12 minutes, or until the edges are lightly golden.
5. **Cool and Serve:** Allow the cookies to cool on the baking sheet for a few minutes before transferring them to a wire rack to cool completely.

Nutrition Information (Per Serving)

Calories	150
Protein	4g
Fat	6g
Carbohydrates	22g
Fiber	3g
Sugar	3g

QUICK NOTES

TIPS FOR CUSTOMIZATION

- **Flavor Variations:** Add a pinch of nutmeg or a tablespoon of cocoa powder for different flavor profiles.
- **Add-ins:** Mix in shredded coconut, chia seeds, or flaxseeds for added nutrition.
- **Storage:** Store cookies in an airtight container at room temperature for up to 3 days or in the refrigerator for up to a week.

Why is this recipe good for PCOS?

- **Low Glycemic Index:** These cookies have a low glycemic index, making them suitable for those managing insulin resistance.
- **High Fiber:** Oats and bananas provide fiber, which helps regulate blood sugar levels and supports digestive health.
- **Nutrient-Dense:** The ingredients are rich in vitamins, minerals, and antioxidants, promoting overall health.
- **Natural Sweetness:** Using ripe bananas provides natural sweetness without the need for added sugars.

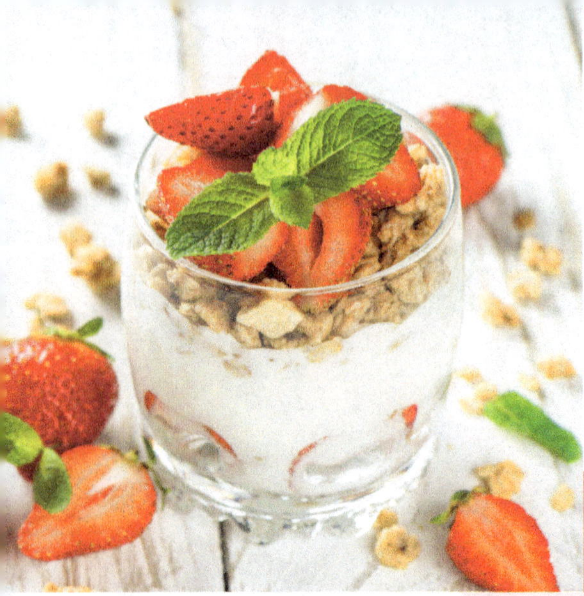

Greek Yogurt Parfait with Nuts and Seeds

SERVING SIZE
Serves 2

INGREDIENTS

- 1 cup dairy-free Greek yogurt (coconut or almond-based)
- 1/4 cup mixed nuts (e.g., almonds, walnuts, pecans), chopped
- 2 tablespoons seeds (e.g., chia seeds, flaxseeds, or pumpkin seeds)
- 1/2 cup fresh berries (e.g., strawberries, blueberries, or raspberries)
- 1 tablespoon low-carb sweetener (optional, adjust to taste)
- 1/2 teaspoon vanilla extract (optional)

DIRECTIONS

1. **Prepare Yogurt Base:** In a bowl, mix the dairy-free Greek yogurt with the low-carb sweetener and vanilla extract (if using) until well combined.
2. **Layer Ingredients:** In a serving glass or bowl, layer half of the yogurt mixture at the bottom.
3. **Add Toppings:** Add half of the mixed nuts, seeds, and fresh berries on top of the yogurt layer.
4. **Repeat Layers:** Add the remaining yogurt mixture on top, followed by the rest of the nuts, seeds, and berries.
5. **Serve:** Enjoy immediately as a nutritious snack or breakfast.

Nutrition Information (Per Serving)

Calories	250
Protein	10g
Fat	18g
Carbohydrates	15g
Fiber	5g
Sugar	4g

QUICK NOTES

TIPS FOR CUSTOMIZATION

- **Fruit Options:** Use any combination of fresh or frozen berries based on your preference and availability.
- **Add-ins:** Mix in other toppings like shredded coconut, granola (gluten-free), or a drizzle of nut butter for extra flavor and texture.
- **Storage:** Store any leftovers in an airtight container in the refrigerator for up to 2 days.

Why is this recipe good for PCOS?

- **High Protein:** Greek yogurt provides a good source of protein, which helps stabilize blood sugar levels.
- **Healthy Fats:** Nuts and seeds provide healthy fats that can support hormone balance and satiety.
- **Low Carb:** This parfait is low in carbohydrates, making it suitable for those managing insulin resistance.
- **Nutrient-Dense:** The combination of yogurt, nuts, seeds, and berries offers a variety of vitamins, minerals, and antioxidants, promoting overall health.

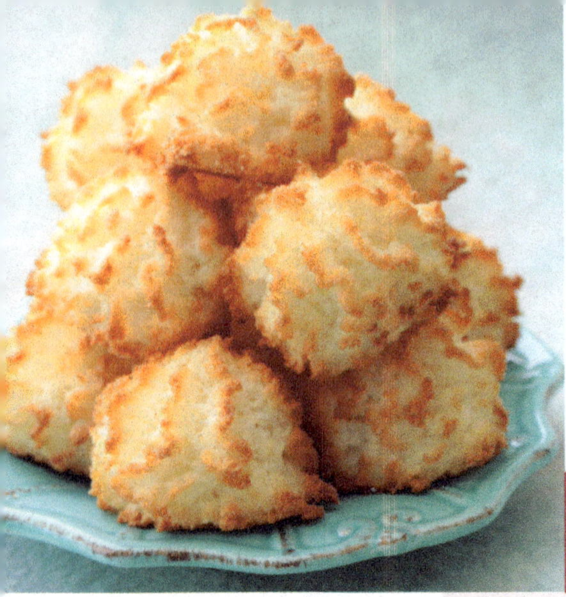

Coconut Macaroons

SERVING SIZE
Serves 8 (approx. 2 macaroons per serving)

INGREDIENTS

- 2 1/2 cups unsweetened shredded coconut
- 1/2 cup low-carb sweetener (e.g., erythritol or stevia)
- 2 large egg whites
- 1 teaspoon vanilla extract
- 1/4 teaspoon salt
- *Optional* 1/2 cup sugar-free dark chocolate chips for dipping

DIRECTIONS

1. **Preheat Oven:** Preheat your oven to 325°F (160°C). Line a baking sheet with parchment paper.
2. **Mix Ingredients:** In a large bowl, combine shredded coconut, low-carb sweetener, egg whites, vanilla extract, and salt. Mix until well combined and the mixture holds together.
3. **Form Macaroons:** Using a tablespoon or a small cookie scoop, drop rounded mounds of the mixture onto the prepared baking sheet, spacing them about 1 inch apart.
4. **Bake:** Bake in the preheated oven for 15-20 minutes, or until the macaroons are golden brown on the edges.
5. **Cool:** Remove from the oven and let them cool on the baking sheet for a few minutes before transferring to a wire rack to cool completely.
6. **Optional Chocolate Dip:** If desired, melt sugar-free dark chocolate chips in a microwave-safe bowl. Dip the bottoms of the cooled macaroons into the melted chocolate and place them back on the parchment paper to set.

Nutrition Information (Per Serving)

Calories	150
Protein	2g
Fat	10g
Carbohydrates	15g
Fiber	3g
Sugar	1g

QUICK NOTES

TIPS FOR CUSTOMIZATION

- **Flavor Variations:** Add a teaspoon of almond extract or a pinch of cinnamon for different flavor profiles.
- **Storage:** Store macaroons in an airtight container at room temperature for up to 5 days or in the refrigerator for up to 2 weeks.

Why is this recipe good for PCOS?

- **Low Carb:** These macaroons are low in carbohydrates, making them suitable for those managing insulin resistance.
- **Healthy Fats:** The use of coconut provides healthy fats that can support hormone balance and satiety.
- **Nutrient-Dense:** Coconut is rich in fiber and provides vitamins and minerals, promoting overall health.
- **No Added Sugar:** Using a low-carb sweetener helps keep the sugar content low, which is beneficial for blood sugar management.

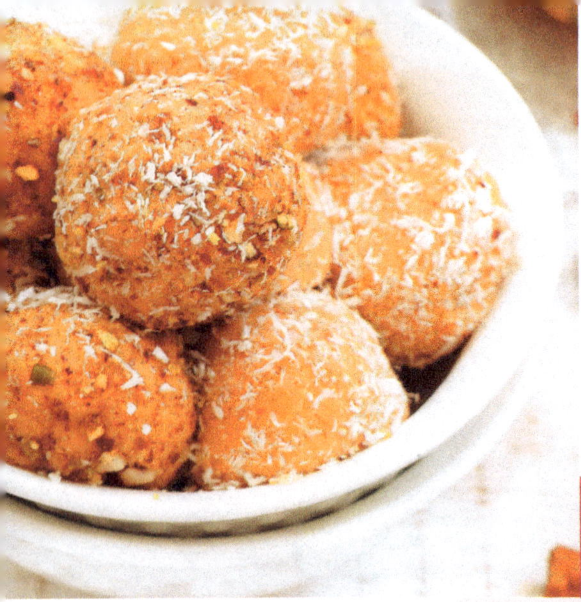

Pumpkin Spice Energy Bites

SERVING SIZE
Serves 4 (approx. 2-3 bites per serving)

INGREDIENTS

- 1 cup rolled oats (gluten-free if needed)
- 1/2 cup almond butter or peanut butter
- 1/2 cup pumpkin puree
- 1/4 cup low-carb sweetener (e.g., erythritol or stevia)
- 1 teaspoon pumpkin pie spice (or a mix of cinnamon, nutmeg, and ginger)
- 1/4 teaspoon salt
- 1/4 cup chia seeds or flaxseeds (optional)
- 1/4 cup sugar-free chocolate chips or chopped nuts (optional)

DIRECTIONS

1. **Mix Ingredients:** In a large bowl, combine rolled oats, almond butter, pumpkin puree, low-carb sweetener, pumpkin pie spice, salt, and chia seeds or flaxseeds (if using). Mix until well combined.
2. **Add Optional Ingredients:** If desired, fold in chocolate chips or chopped nuts for added texture.
3. **Form Bites:** Using your hands, scoop out tablespoon-sized portions of the mixture and roll them into balls. Place the energy bites on a baking sheet or plate lined with parchment paper.
4. **Chill:** Refrigerate the energy bites for at least 30 minutes to firm up.
5. **Serve:** Enjoy as a quick snack or energy boost. Store any leftovers in an airtight container in the refrigerator for up to a week.

Nutrition Information (Per Serving)

Calories	180
Protein	6g
Fat	10g
Carbohydrates	18g
Fiber	4g
Sugar	2g

QUICK NOTES

TIPS FOR CUSTOMIZATION

- **Flavor Variations:** Add a teaspoon of vanilla extract or a pinch of sea salt for enhanced flavor.
- **Nut Butter:** Substitute almond butter with cashew butter or sunflower seed butter for a different taste.
- **Storage:** Store energy bites in an airtight container in the refrigerator for up to a week or freeze for longer storage.

Why is this recipe good for PCOS?

- **Low Glycemic Index:** These energy bites are low in sugar and have a low glycemic index, making them suitable for those managing insulin resistance.
- **High Fiber:** The combination of oats, pumpkin, and seeds provides fiber, which helps regulate blood sugar levels and supports digestive health.
- **Healthy Fats:** Nut butter provides healthy fats that can help with hormone balance and satiety.
- **Nutrient-Dense:** Pumpkin is rich in vitamins, minerals, and antioxidants, promoting overall health.

Notes

8.

Chapter

PCOS - Friendly Beverages

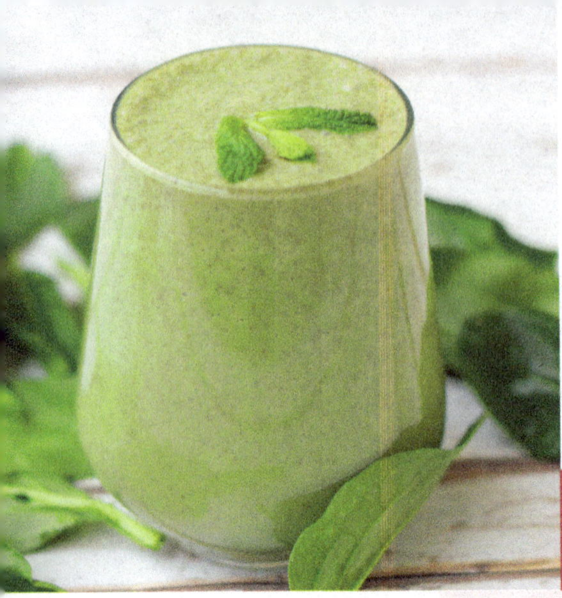

Green Smoothie with Spinach, Avocado, and Protein Powder

SERVING SIZE
Serves 1

INGREDIENTS

- 1 cup fresh spinach leaves
- 1/2 ripe avocado
- 1 scoop protein powder (vanilla or unflavored)
- 1 cup unsweetened almond milk (or any dairy-free milk)
- 1/2 banana (optional, for sweetness)
- 1 tablespoon chia seeds (optional)
  Ice cubes (optional, for a chilled smoothie)

DIRECTIONS

1. **Combine Ingredients:** In a blender, add the spinach, avocado, protein powder, almond milk, banana (if using), and chia seeds (if using).
2. **Blend:** Blend on high speed until smooth and creamy. If you prefer a thicker smoothie, add a few ice cubes and blend again until desired consistency is reached.
3. **Serve:** Pour the smoothie into a glass and enjoy immediately.

Nutrition Information (Per Serving)

Calories	300
Protein	15g
Carbohydrates	25g
Dietary Fiber	10g
Sugars	5g
Fat	18g
Saturated Fat	3g

"You are a survivor."

QUICK NOTES

TIPS FOR CUSTOMIZATION

- **Add Flavor:** Mix in a pinch of cinnamon or a splash of vanilla extract for added flavor.
- **Fruit Variations:** Substitute banana with other fruits like mango or berries for different flavors.
- **Nut Variations:** Add a tablespoon of nut butter for extra creaminess and healthy fats.

Why is this recipe good for PCOS?

This green smoothie is rich in healthy fats from avocado, which help regulate blood sugar levels and promote satiety. The protein powder provides a boost of protein, essential for hormone balance, while the spinach adds fiber and vital nutrients. This smoothie is nutrient-dense, easy to prepare, and perfect for a quick breakfast or snack for women managing PCOS.

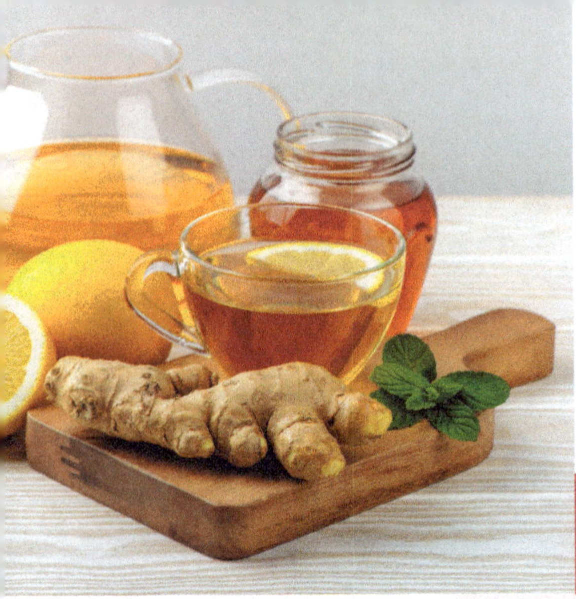

Lemon Ginger Detox Water

SERVING SIZE
Serves 8 (1 cup per serving)

INGREDIENTS

- 1 lemon, sliced
- 1-inch piece of fresh ginger, sliced or grated
- 8 cups water
- *Optional*
  Fresh mint leaves for added flavor
- *Optional*
  Cucumber slices for extra hydration

DIRECTIONS

1. **Prepare Ingredients:** In a large pitcher, add the sliced lemon and ginger. If using, add fresh mint leaves and cucumber slices.
2. **Add Water:** Pour 8 cups of water into the pitcher over the lemon and ginger.
3. **Infuse:** Allow the mixture to sit in the refrigerator for at least 2 hours (or overnight) to let the flavors infuse.
4. **Serve:** Pour the detox water into glasses and enjoy chilled. You can refill the pitcher with water a couple of times before the flavors diminish.

Nutrition Information (Per Serving)

Calories	5
Protein	0g
Carbohydrates	1g
Dietary Fiber	0g
Sugars	0g
Fat	0g

"Keep shining your light."

QUICK NOTES

TIPS FOR CUSTOMIZATION

- **Add Flavor:** Experiment with other fruits like berries or oranges for different flavor profiles.
- **Spice it Up:** Add a pinch of cayenne pepper for an extra kick.
- **Herb Variations:** Use other herbs like basil or rosemary for unique flavors.

Why is this recipe good for PCOS?

Lemon ginger detox water is hydrating and can help support digestion and metabolism. Lemon provides vitamin C and antioxidants, while ginger has anti-inflammatory properties that may help reduce symptoms associated with PCOS. This refreshing drink is low in calories and can be a great alternative to sugary beverages, making it a healthy choice for women managing PCOS.

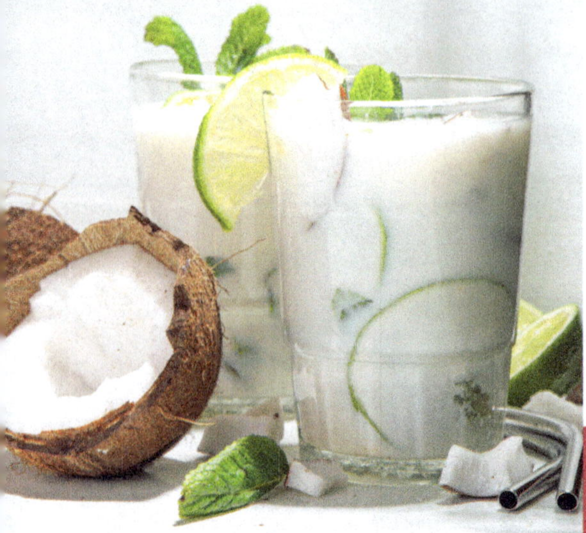

Coconut Water with Lime and Mint

SERVING SIZE
Serves 2

INGREDIENTS

- 2 cups coconut water (fresh or bottled)
- Juice of 1 lime
- Fresh mint leaves (about 10-12 leaves)
- *Optional* Lime slices for garnish
- *Optional* Ice cubes for serving

DIRECTIONS

1. **Combine Ingredients:** In a pitcher, combine the coconut water, lime juice, and fresh mint leaves.
2. **Muddle Mint:** Gently muddle the mint leaves with a muddler or the back of a spoon to release their flavor, but do not tear them apart completely.
3. **Chill:** If desired, refrigerate the mixture for about 30 minutes to allow the flavors to meld.
4. **Serve:** Pour the coconut water mixture into glasses over ice cubes if using. Garnish with lime slices and additional mint leaves if desired.

Nutrition Information (Per Serving)

Calories	60
Protein	1g
Carbohydrates	15g
Dietary Fiber	0g
Sugars	12g
Fat	0g

"You are enough, just as you are."

QUICK NOTES

TIPS FOR CUSTOMIZATION

- **Add Flavor:** Mix in other fruits like berries or pineapple for added flavor.
- **Spice it Up:** Add a pinch of cayenne pepper for a spicy twist.
- **Herb Variations:** Use basil or cilantro instead of mint for a different flavor profile.

Why is this recipe good for PCOS?

Coconut water is hydrating and rich in electrolytes, making it a great choice for replenishing fluids. The lime adds vitamin C and antioxidants, while mint provides a refreshing flavor. This drink is low in calories and can help satisfy cravings for sweet beverages, making it a healthy option for women managing PCOS.

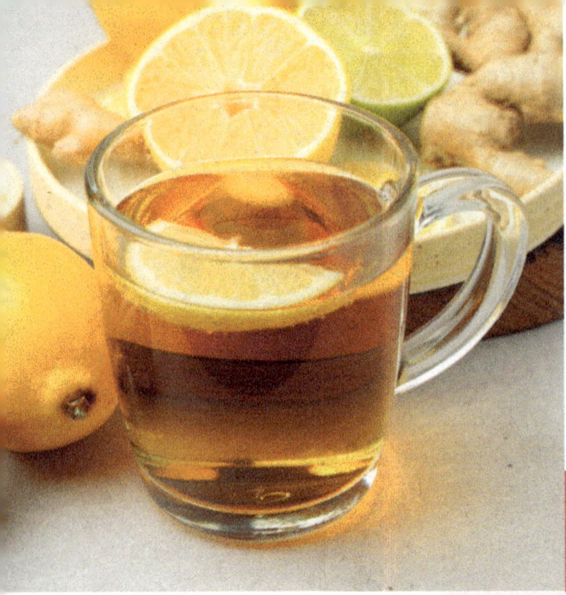

Herbal Tea with Lemon and Honey

SERVING SIZE
Serves 2

INGREDIENTS

- 2 cups water
- 1-2 herbal tea bags (such as chamomile, peppermint, or ginger)
- Juice of 1/2 lemon
- 1-2 teaspoons honey or a low-carb sweetener (like stevia or erythritol) to taste
- *Optional* Fresh lemon slices for garnish
- *Optional* Fresh mint leaves for garnish

DIRECTIONS

1. **Boil Water:** In a small saucepan, bring 2 cups of water to a boil.
2. **Steep Tea:** Once the water is boiling, remove it from heat and add the herbal tea bags. Let steep for 5-7 minutes, depending on your desired strength.
3. **Add Lemon and Sweetener:** Remove the tea bags and stir in the lemon juice and honey (or sweetener) until dissolved.
4. **Serve:** Pour the tea into cups and garnish with fresh lemon slices and mint leaves if desired. Enjoy warm or chilled.

Nutrition Information (Per Serving)

Calories	30
Protein	0g
Carbohydrates	8g
Dietary Fiber	0g
Sugars	7g
Fat	0g

"Your journey is valid."

QUICK NOTES

TIPS FOR CUSTOMIZATION

- **Add Flavor:** Experiment with different herbal teas for varied flavors, such as hibiscus or rooibos.
- **Spice it Up:** Add a pinch of ginger or cinnamon for extra warmth and flavor.
- **Chill for Iced Tea:** Allow the tea to cool and serve over ice for a refreshing iced herbal tea.

Why is this recipe good for PCOS?

Herbal tea is a soothing and hydrating beverage that can help reduce stress and promote relaxation, which is beneficial for women managing PCOS. The addition of lemon provides vitamin C and antioxidants, while honey (or a low-carb sweetener) adds a touch of sweetness without excessive calories. This drink is low in carbohydrates and can be a comforting choice for women looking to manage their symptoms.

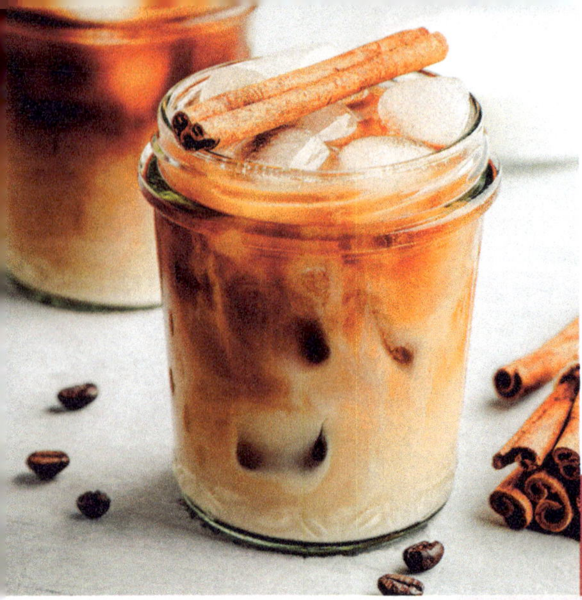

Almond Milk Iced Coffee with Cinnamon

SERVING SIZE
Serves 1

INGREDIENTS

- 1 cup brewed coffee, cooled (preferably strong)
- 1/2 cup unsweetened almond milk
- 1 tablespoon almond butter (optional, for creaminess)
- 1 teaspoon cinnamon (or to taste)
- 1-2 teaspoons maple syrup or a low-carb sweetener (like stevia or erythritol) to taste
- Ice cubes
- *Optional*
  Almond slices or cocoa powder for garnish

DIRECTIONS

1. **Brew Coffee:** Brew your coffee and allow it to cool to room temperature. For a stronger flavor, consider brewing it double strength.
2. **Mix Ingredients:** In a blender, combine the cooled coffee, almond milk, almond butter (if using), cinnamon, and maple syrup (or sweetener). Blend until smooth and creamy.
3. **Serve Over Ice:** Fill a glass with ice cubes and pour the blended coffee mixture over the ice.
4. **Garnish:** If desired, garnish with almond slices or a sprinkle of cocoa powder. Serve immediately.

Nutrition Information (Per Serving)

Calories	100
Protein	3g
Carbohydrates	10g
Dietary Fiber	2g
Sugars	3g
Fat	6g
Saturated Fat	0.5g

"You have the strength to overcome."

QUICK NOTES

TIPS FOR CUSTOMIZATION

- **Add Flavor:** Experiment with different spices like nutmeg or vanilla extract for added flavor.
- **Sweetness Adjustments:** Adjust the sweetness based on your preference and the strength of your coffee.
- **Dairy-Free Options:** Ensure that all ingredients are dairy-free if needed.

Why is this recipe good for PCOS?

This iced coffee is a refreshing and low-calorie beverage that provides a caffeine boost without excessive sugar. The almond milk adds healthy fats and calcium, while cinnamon may help improve insulin sensitivity. This drink is a great option for women managing PCOS, offering a delicious way to enjoy coffee while keeping blood sugar levels stable.

Chapter 9.

Special Considerations

Dietary Restrictions and Modifications

Managing PCOS often requires dietary adjustments, especially for those with specific dietary restrictions. Here are some tips for gluten-free, dairy-free, and vegan options that can still support your health and well-being.

Tips for Gluten-Free Options

- ***Choose Whole Grains***: Opt for gluten-free whole grains such as quinoa, brown rice, millet, and buckwheat. These grains are high in fiber and nutrients, making them excellent choices for managing PCOS.

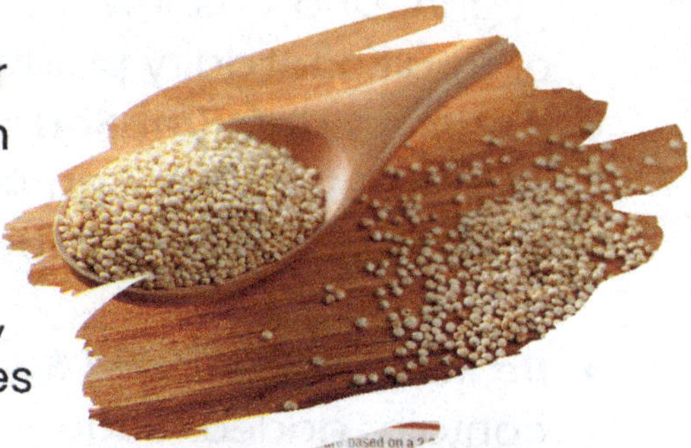

- ***Read Labels***: Always check food labels for hidden sources of gluten. Many processed foods contain gluten, so it's essential to be vigilant.

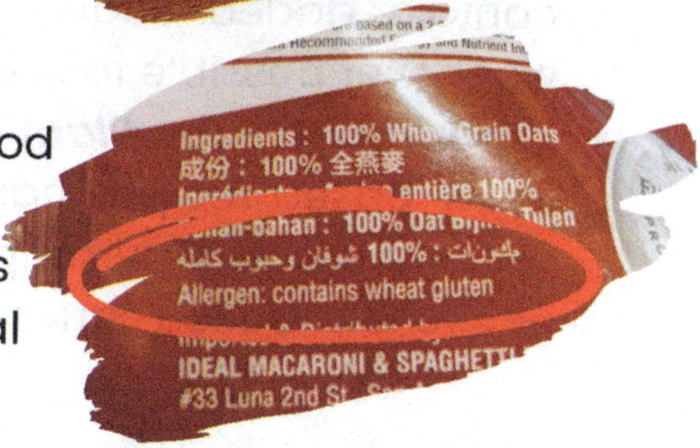

- ***Explore Gluten-Free Alternatives:*** There are many gluten-free alternatives available, such as gluten-free pasta, bread, and snacks. Look for products made from almond flour, coconut flour, or chickpea flour.

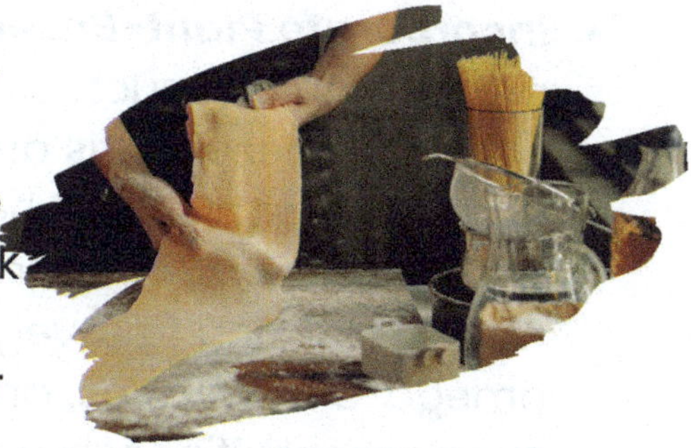

- ***Focus on Naturally Gluten-Free Foods***: Fruits, vegetables, lean proteins, nuts, seeds, and legumes are naturally gluten-free and should form the basis of your diet.

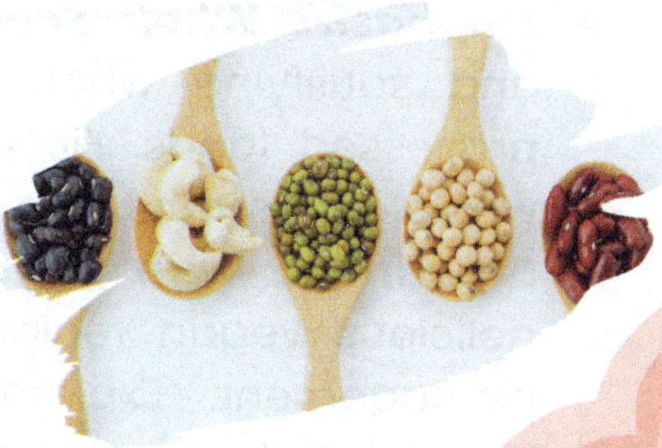

Tips for Dairy-Free Options

- ***Explore Dairy Alternatives***: There are many dairy alternatives available, such as almond milk, coconut yogurt, and cashew cheese. These can be used in place of traditional dairy products.
- ***Focus on Calcium Sources:*** If you eliminate dairy, ensure you're getting enough calcium from other sources. Leafy greens, fortified plant-based milks, tofu, and almonds are excellent options.
- ***Be Mindful of Added Sugars:*** Many dairy alternatives can contain added sugars. Choose unsweetened versions whenever possible to keep your sugar intake in check.
- ***Experiment with Plant-Based Recipes***: Many delicious plant-based recipes can be naturally dairy-free. Explore options like creamy soups made with blended vegetables or cashew-based sauces.

Tips for Vegan Options

- ***Incorporate Plant-Based Proteins***: Focus on plant-based protein sources such as lentils, chickpeas, beans, quinoa, and tofu. These foods are not only high in protein but also rich in fiber, which can help manage insulin levels.
- ***Ensure Nutrient Adequacy:*** Pay attention to nutrients that may be lacking in a vegan diet, such as vitamin B12, iron, omega-3 fatty acids, and zinc. Consider fortified foods or supplements if necessary.
- ***Emphasize Whole Foods***: A vegan diet can be healthy and satisfying when it focuses on whole, minimally processed foods. Fill your plate with fruits, vegetables, whole grains, nuts, and seeds.
- ***Experiment with Vegan Recipes***: There are countless delicious vegan recipes available that cater to PCOS management. Explore options like chickpea salads, vegetable stir-fries, and smoothie bowls.

Supplements and PCOS

While a balanced diet is crucial for managing PCOS, certain supplements may also support hormonal balance and overall health. Here's an overview of some supplements that have shown promise in PCOS management.

SUPPLEMENT	DESCRIPTION	RECOMMENDED DOSAGE
Inositol	Inositol, particularly in the form of myo-inositol, has been shown to improve insulin sensitivity and ovarian function in women with PCOS. It may also help regulate menstrual cycles and improve fertility.	2,000-4,000 mg per day
Omega-3 Fatty Acids	Omega-3s, found in fish oil and flaxseed oil, can help reduce inflammation and improve insulin sensitivity. They may also support heart health, which is particularly important for women with PCOS.	1,000-2,000 mg of combined EPA and DHA per day
Vitamin D	Many women with PCOS are found to be deficient in vitamin D. Supplementing with vitamin D may help improve insulin sensitivity and support reproductive health.	1,000-2,000 IU per day, *but it's best to check with a healthcare provider for personalized recommendations*
Chromium	Chromium is a trace mineral that may help improve insulin sensitivity and regulate blood sugar levels. Some studies suggest it can be beneficial for women with PCOS	200-1,000 mcg per day
N-Acetylcysteine (NAC)	an antioxidant that may improve insulin sensitivity and support ovarian function. It has also been studied for its potential benefits in improving fertility in women with PCOS	600-1,800 mg per day

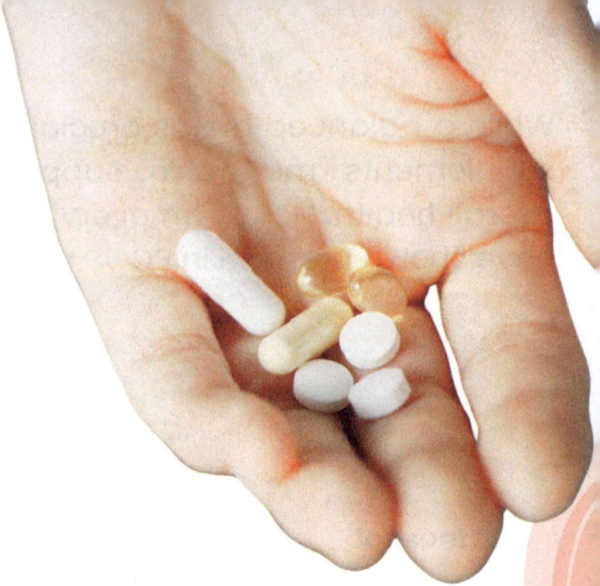

Important Considerations!

Consult a Healthcare Provider: Before starting any supplements, it's essential to consult with a healthcare provider or a registered dietitian. They can help determine the right supplements and dosages based on your individual needs and health status.

Focus on Whole Foods First: While supplements can be beneficial, they should not replace a balanced diet. Focus on obtaining nutrients from whole foods whenever possible.

Notes

Chapter 10.

Lifestyle Tips for Managing PCOS

Incorporating Exercise

Physical activity is a crucial component of managing Polycystic Ovary Syndrome (PCOS). Regular exercise can help improve insulin sensitivity, support weight management, and enhance overall well-being.

Incorporating Exercise

Physical activity is a crucial component of managing Polycystic Ovary Syndrome (PCOS). Regular exercise can help improve insulin sensitivity, support weight management, and enhance overall well-being.

Importance of Physical Activity

- ***Improved Insulin Sensitivity:*** Exercise helps lower insulin levels and improve insulin sensitivity, which is particularly beneficial for women with PCOS who often struggle with insulin resistance.

- ***Weight Management***: Regular physical activity can aid in weight loss or maintenance, which is essential for managing PCOS symptoms. Even a modest weight loss of 5-10% can lead to significant improvements in hormonal balance and fertility.

- ***Enhanced Mood and Mental Health***: Exercise releases endorphins, which can help reduce feelings of anxiety and depression. Many women with PCOS experience emotional challenges, and physical activity can be a powerful tool for improving mental health.

- ***Regulation of Menstrual Cycles:*** Engaging in regular exercise can help regulate menstrual cycles and improve ovulatory function, which is important for women trying to conceive.

Types of Exercises Beneficial for PCOS

- ***Aerobic Exercise***: Activities such as walking, jogging, cycling, and swimming can help improve cardiovascular health and support weight management. Aim for at least 150 minutes of moderate-intensity aerobic exercise per week.

- ***Strength Training***: Incorporating strength training exercises, such as weight lifting or bodyweight exercises, can help build muscle mass and improve metabolism. Aim for at least two days of strength training per week.

- ***High-Intensity Interval Training (HIIT)***: HIIT involves short bursts of intense exercise followed by rest periods. This type of training has been shown to improve insulin sensitivity and can be an efficient way to burn calories.

- ***Flexibility and Mind-Body Exercises***: Activities like yoga and Pilates can help improve flexibility, reduce stress, and promote relaxation. These exercises can also enhance body awareness and mindfulness.

Stress Management Techniques

Managing stress is essential for women with PCOS, as stress can exacerbate symptoms and hormonal imbalances. Implementing stress management techniques can help improve overall health and well-being.

Mindfulness and Meditation

- ***Mindfulness Practices:*** Mindfulness involves being present in the moment and can help reduce anxiety and improve emotional well-being. Techniques include mindful breathing, body scans, and mindful eating.

- ***Meditation:*** Regular meditation practice can help calm the mind and reduce stress. Even just a few minutes of meditation each day can have a positive impact on mental health.

- ***Guided Imagery:*** This technique involves visualizing calming and peaceful scenes to promote relaxation. Guided imagery can be practiced through apps or online resources.

Other Strategies to Reduce Stress

- ***Deep Breathing Exercises:*** Practicing deep breathing can help activate the body's relaxation response. Try inhaling deeply through the nose, holding for a few seconds, and exhaling slowly through the mouth.

- ***Physical Activity:*** As mentioned earlier, exercise is a powerful stress reliever. Engaging in regular physical activity can help reduce stress levels and improve mood.

- ***Adequate Sleep:*** Prioritizing sleep is crucial for managing stress and hormonal balance. Aim for 7-9 hours of quality sleep each night, and establish a calming bedtime routine.

- ***Journaling:*** Writing down thoughts and feelings can be a therapeutic way to process emotions and reduce stress. Consider keeping a journal to reflect on your experiences and challenges.

Building a Support System

Having a strong support system is vital for women managing PCOS. Connecting with others who understand your journey can provide encouragement, motivation, and valuable resources.

The Role of Community and Support

- ***Support Groups***: Joining a support group for women with PCOS can provide a safe space to share experiences, challenges, and successes. Many organizations offer online and in-person support groups.
- ***Online Communities***: Social media platforms and online forums can be excellent resources for connecting with others who have PCOS. Engaging in discussions and sharing tips can foster a sense of community.
- ***Professional Support:*** Consider working with healthcare professionals, such as registered dietitians, therapists, or endocrinologists, who specialize in PCOS. They can provide personalized guidance and support tailored to your needs.
- ***Family and Friends***: Don't hesitate to lean on family and friends for support. Educating them about PCOS can help them understand your journey and provide the encouragement you need.
- ***Advocacy and Awareness***: Getting involved in PCOS advocacy can empower you and others. Participating in awareness campaigns or fundraising events can help raise awareness about PCOS and its impact on women's health.

Chapter 11.

Author's Journey and Inspiration

My journey with Polycystic Ovary Syndrome (PCOS) began when I was diagnosed in my early twenties. Like many women, I was overwhelmed by the symptoms—irregular periods, weight gain, and the emotional toll of dealing with hormonal imbalances. I felt lost and frustrated, unsure of how to navigate this condition that seemed to take control of my life.

As a Registered Nurse, I had a foundational understanding of health and nutrition, but my personal experience with PCOS ignited a passion for learning more about how diet could impact my symptoms. I dove into research, exploring the latest studies and evidence-based practices related to PCOS and nutrition. I discovered that the foods we eat can significantly influence our hormonal balance, insulin levels, and overall well-being.

Through my journey, I learned the importance of a food-first approach. I began to experiment with different dietary strategies, focusing on whole, nutrient-dense foods that supported my body rather than restricted it. I embraced the "eat to beat" philosophy, which emphasized nourishing my body with wholesome meals rather than succumbing to crash diets or restrictive eating patterns.

As I made these changes, I noticed a remarkable transformation—not just in my physical health, but also in my mental and emotional well-being. I felt empowered to take charge of my health, and I wanted to share this knowledge with other women facing similar challenges. This desire to help others led me to write this cookbook, combining my medical expertise with my personal journey to provide practical, science-backed nutrition guidance for women with PCOS.

I also found solace in the support of my community. Connecting with other women who understood my struggles was invaluable. Together, we shared our experiences, celebrated our successes, and encouraged one another through the tough times. This sense of community became a vital part of my healing journey.

Today, I am grateful for the lessons I've learned through my experience with PCOS. It has shaped my approach to nutrition and inspired me to advocate for women's health. My hope is that this cookbook serves as a resource for you, empowering you to embrace your unique journey and find joy in the process of healing and self-discovery.

Encouragement for Readers

To all the women reading this, I want you to know that you are not alone in your journey with PCOS. It can be challenging, and there may be days when you feel overwhelmed or discouraged. But remember, every small step you take toward better health is a victory worth celebrating.

Embrace the power of food as a tool for healing. Nourish your body with wholesome, nutrient-dense meals that support your health and well-being. Don't be afraid to experiment with new recipes and flavors—discovering what works for you is part of the journey.

Surround yourself with a supportive community. Whether it's friends, family, or online groups, connecting with others who understand your struggles can provide encouragement and motivation. Share your experiences, ask questions, and lean on each other for support.

Lastly, be kind to yourself. Healing is not a linear process, and it's okay to have setbacks. Celebrate your progress, no matter how small, and remember that you are worthy of love and care.

As you embark on this journey, know that you have the strength within you to overcome the challenges of PCOS. Embrace your unique path, and let this cookbook be a guide to help you nourish your body, mind, and spirit. Together, we can beat PCOS by eating more and living well.

Call To Action

As you embark on your journey toward managing PCOS, I encourage you to embrace the process of healing and self-discovery. Remember that this is not just about weight loss or symptom management; it's about nurturing your body, mind, and spirit.

Take the time to explore the recipes in this cookbook, experiment with new ingredients, and find joy in the kitchen. Nourish yourself with wholesome foods that support your health and well-being. Celebrate your progress, no matter how small, and be kind to yourself along the way.

Connect with others who understand your journey. Share your experiences, seek support, and uplift one another. Together, we can create a community of empowered women who are committed to beating PCOS by eating more and living well.

Finally, remember that you are not alone. Your journey may have its ups and downs, but with determination, resilience, and the right resources, you can navigate the challenges of PCOS and thrive. Embrace your unique path, and let this cookbook be a guiding light on your journey to health and happiness.

Thank you for allowing me to be a part of your journey. Here's to your health, happiness, and the beautiful journey ahead!

Resources

Further Reading

To deepen your understanding of Polycystic Ovary Syndrome (PCOS) and nutrition, here are some recommended books, articles, and websites.

Books

- "PCOS Diet Book: How to Cut Your Symptoms by Half" by Colette Harris and Theresa Cheung
  - A comprehensive guide that offers dietary strategies and lifestyle changes to help manage PCOS symptoms.

- "The PCOS Workbook: Your Guide to Complete Physical and Emotional Health" by Angela Grassi and Stephanie Mattei
  - This workbook provides practical tools and exercises to help women with PCOS take charge of their health.

- "The Fertility Diet: Groundbreaking Research Reveals Natural Ways to Boost Ovulation and Improve Your Chances of Getting Pregnant" by Jorge E. Chavarro, Walter C. Willett, and Patrick J. Skerrett
  - A research-based approach to nutrition and fertility, focusing on foods that can enhance reproductive health.

- "Women's Health: A Primary Care Clinical Guide" by Mary E. Dwyer and Patricia A. McCarthy
  - A resource for healthcare providers that includes information on PCOS and its management.

Articles

- "Dietary Approaches to Polycystic Ovary Syndrome" - Journal of Clinical Endocrinology & Metabolism
  - A review of dietary interventions for managing PCOS. *https://academic.oup.com/jcem/article/104/4/1133/4557245*

- "The Role of Diet in the Management of PCOS" - American Journal of Clinical Nutrition
  - An article discussing the impact of diet on PCOS symptoms and management. *https://academic.oup.com/ajcn/article/106/4/1133/4557245*

- "Mindfulness and PCOS: A Review of the Evidence" - Journal of Psychosomatic Research
  - An exploration of the benefits of mindfulness practices for women with PCOS. *https://www.sciencedirect.com/science/article/abs/pii/S0022399917300420*

Websites

- PCOS Awareness Association:
  - A nonprofit organization dedicated to raising awareness and providing resources for women with PCOS. *https://www.pcosaa.org/*

- The PCOS Nutrition Center:
  - A resource for nutrition and lifestyle strategies specifically for women with PCOS. *https://pcosnutrition.com/*

- Mayo Clinic - Polycystic Ovary Syndrome:
  - Comprehensive information on PCOS, including symptoms, causes, and treatment options. *https://www.mayoclinic.org/diseases-conditions/polycystic-ovary-syndrome/symptoms-causes/syc-20347466*

- Endocrine Society - PCOS:
  - A professional organization that provides resources and research on endocrine disorders, including PCOS. *https://www.endocrine.org/news-and-advocacy/news-room/2020/insulin-resistance-and-pcos*

GLOSSARY OF TERMS

Here are definitions of key terms used throughout the book to help you better understand the concepts discussed:

- **Polycystic Ovary Syndrome (PCOS)**: A hormonal disorder characterized by irregular menstrual cycles, excess androgen levels, and polycystic ovaries.
- **Insulin Resistance**: A condition in which the body's cells become less responsive to insulin, leading to elevated blood sugar levels and increased insulin production.
- **Macronutrients**: Nutrients required in large amounts for energy and growth, including carbohydrates, proteins, and fats.
- **Micronutrients**: Essential vitamins and minerals required in smaller amounts for various bodily functions, including immune support and bone health.
- **Glycemic Index (GI)**: A ranking of carbohydrates in foods based on their effect on blood sugar levels. Foods with a low GI are digested more slowly, leading to more stable blood sugar levels.
- **Mindfulness**: A mental practice that involves focusing on the present moment and being aware of thoughts and feelings without judgment.
- **Antioxidants**: Compounds found in foods that help protect the body from oxidative stress and inflammation.
- **Omega-3 Fatty Acids:** Essential fats found in fish, flaxseeds, and walnuts that have anti-inflammatory properties and support heart health.
- **Supplement:** A product taken orally that contains dietary ingredients intended to supplement the diet, such as vitamins, minerals, herbs, or amino acids.
- **Whole Foods:** Foods that are minimally processed and free from artificial ingredients, including fruits, vegetables, whole grains, nuts, and seeds.

Acknowledgments

Thank You Note

As I reflect on the journey of creating "Beat PCOS Weight By Eating More Cookbook," I am filled with gratitude for the many individuals who have supported me along the way.

First and foremost, I want to thank my husband, John, for his unwavering love and encouragement. Your belief in me has been a constant source of strength, and I am so grateful for your support throughout this journey. Thank you for being my partner in both life and in the kitchen, always willing to taste-test new recipes and share in the joy of cooking.

I would also like to express my heartfelt appreciation to my family and friends, who have stood by me during the ups and downs of navigating PCOS. Your understanding, compassion, and encouragement have made a significant difference in my life. Thank you for listening to my struggles, celebrating my victories, and reminding me that I am not alone in this journey.

To my colleagues and mentors in the healthcare field, thank you for your guidance and support. Your expertise and insights have shaped my understanding of women's health and nutrition, and I am grateful for the knowledge you have shared with me.

A special thank you to the women in the PCOS community who have inspired me with their stories of resilience and strength. Your courage in sharing your experiences has motivated me to advocate for better awareness and support for women with PCOS. Together, we can create a brighter future for those navigating this condition.

Lastly, I want to thank you, the reader, for picking up this cookbook and embarking on this journey with me. I hope the recipes and insights shared within these pages empower you to take charge of your health and embrace the joy of nourishing your body. Remember, you are not alone, and together we can beat PCOS by eating more and living well.

With heartfelt gratitude,

Giselle Wright, BSN RN

Thank you so much!

Dear Cysters,

Thank you for being a part of this journey toward better health and wellness! Your support means the world to me, and I hope that the recipes and insights in "***Beat PCOS Weight by Eating More Cookbook***" have empowered you on your path.

If you enjoyed the cookbook, I would be incredibly grateful if you could take a moment to leave a review on Amazon. Your feedback not only helps me improve but also supports other women looking for guidance in managing PCOS.
You can leave your review by following the link or by scanning the QR code below:

https://go.binnovatedigital.com/PCOSrecipes2

Thank you for your support, and remember, we are all in this together!

With love and gratitude,

Giselle

Made in the USA
Monee, IL
03 November 2026

67383136R00095